Check out these video tutorials I made for the book! I hope this playlist will help you. Also, if you like, could you share how the book and videos worked for you? Thanks in advance!

Scan the QR code to watch the videos!

Do you have problem accessing the videos? Email me at avfitness99coaching@gmail.com and I'll sort it for you.

Contents

INTRODUCTION 1

HOW TO READ THE BOOK FOR BEST RESULTS 3

CHAIR YOGA STRETCHES 4

CHAIR YOGA STRENGTHENING 12

CHAIR YOGA CARDIO 21

28-DAY PLAN 33

CONCLUSION 63

Disclaimer

The information provided in this book is intended far educational and informational purposes only. It is not a substitute far professional medicai advice, diagnosis, or treatment. Always seek the advice of your physician or other qualified healthcare provider before starting any new fitness program or making any changes to an existing one. The author and publisher of this book are not responsible far any injury or health problems that may result from the use of the information in this book.

CHAIR YOGA STRETCHES

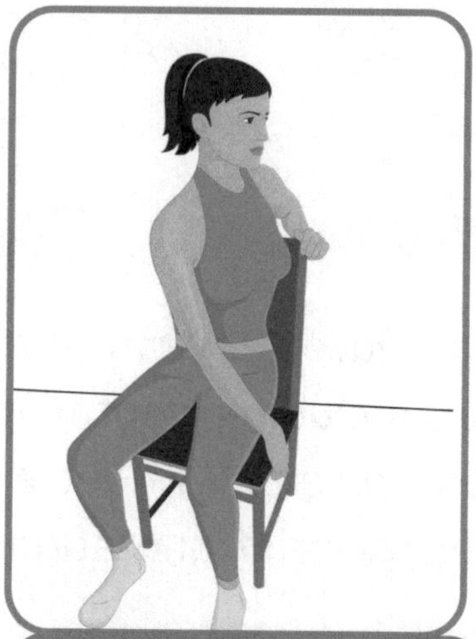

Chair Twist

Pag 04

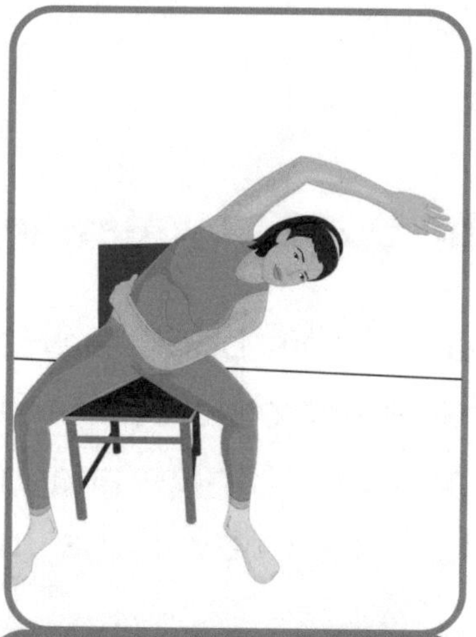

Chair Side Opening

Pag 05

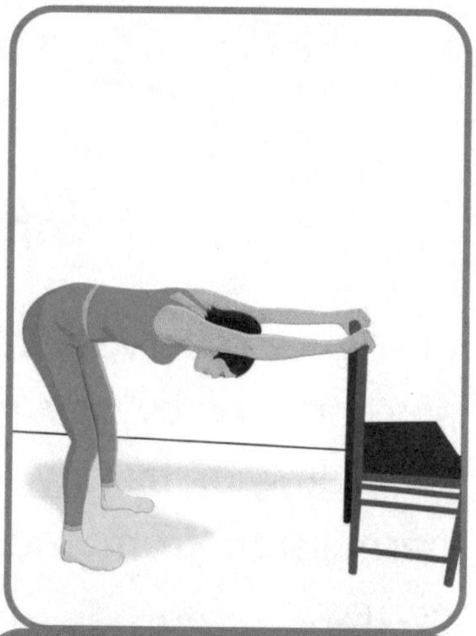

Chair Back Stretch

Pag 06

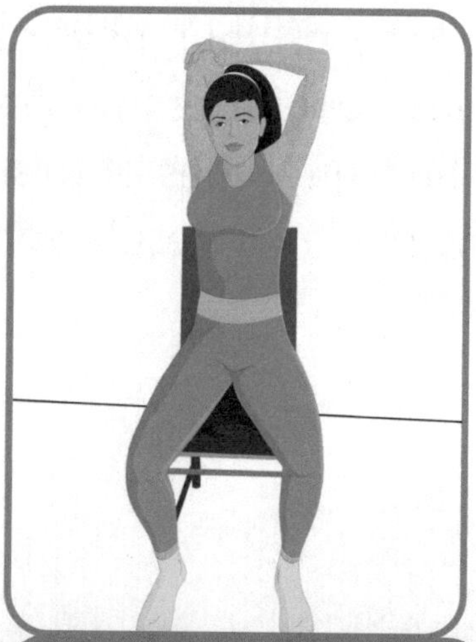

Chair Triceps Stretch

Pag 07

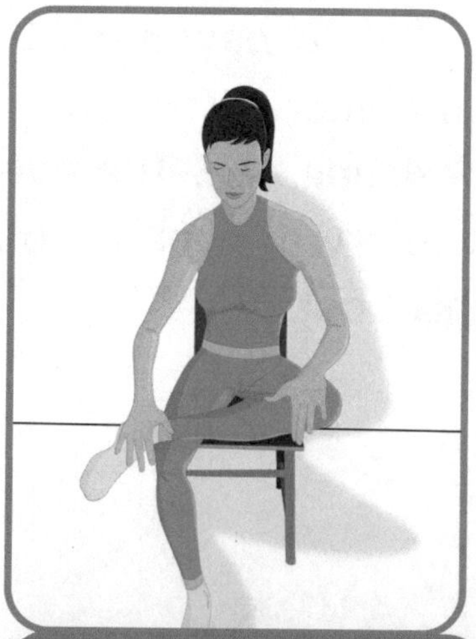

Chair Glute Stretch

Pag 08

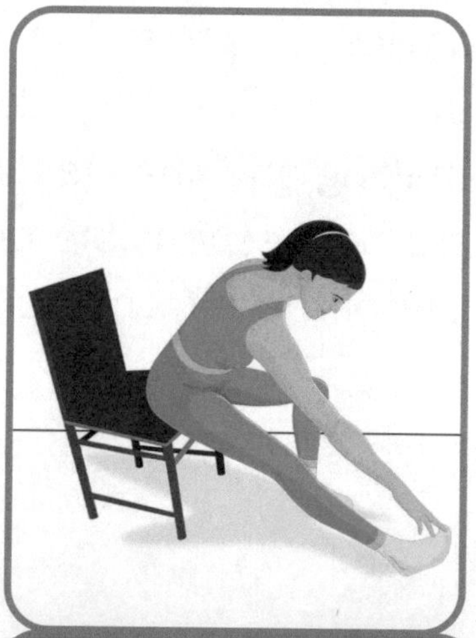

Chair Calf Stretch

Pag 09

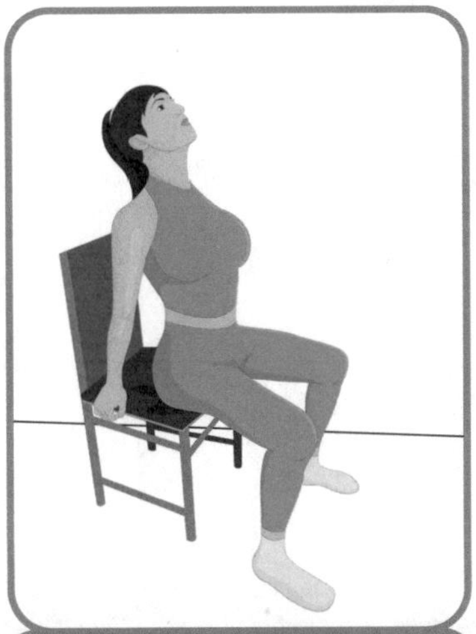

Chair Opening Chest

Pag 10

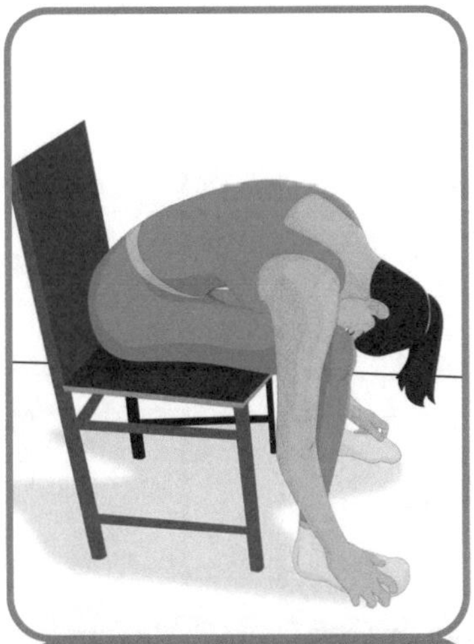

Chair Forward Fold

Pag 11

CHAIR YOGA STRENGTHENING

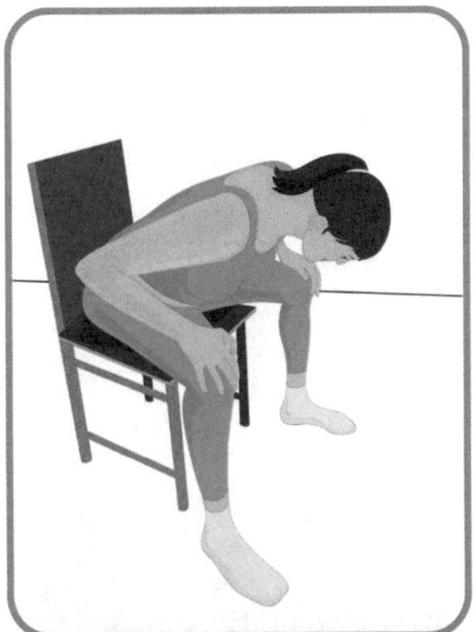

Chair Push Up

Pag 12

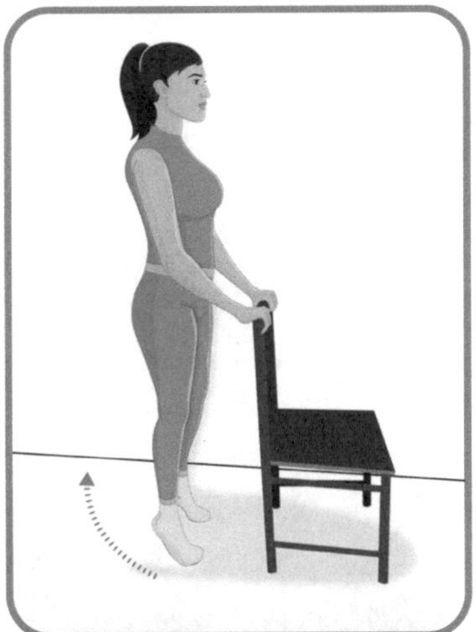

Chair Calf Raises

Pag 13

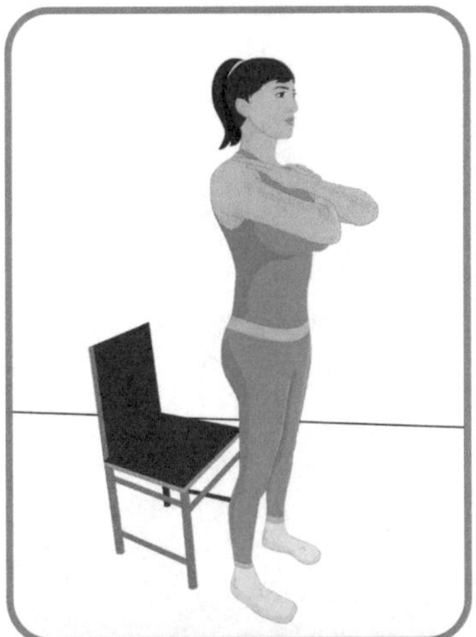

Chair Squat

Pag 14

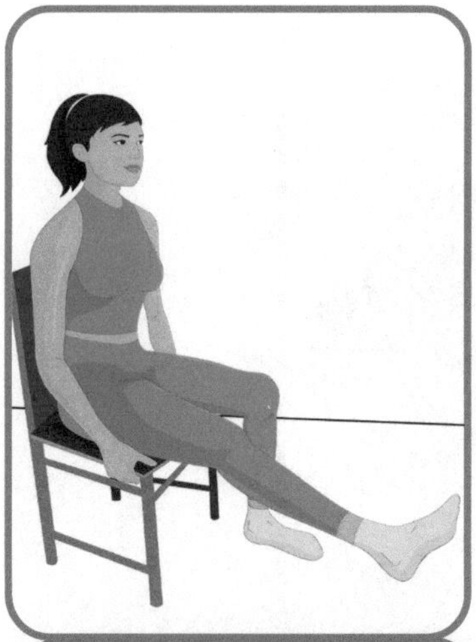

Chair Leg Extension
Pag 15

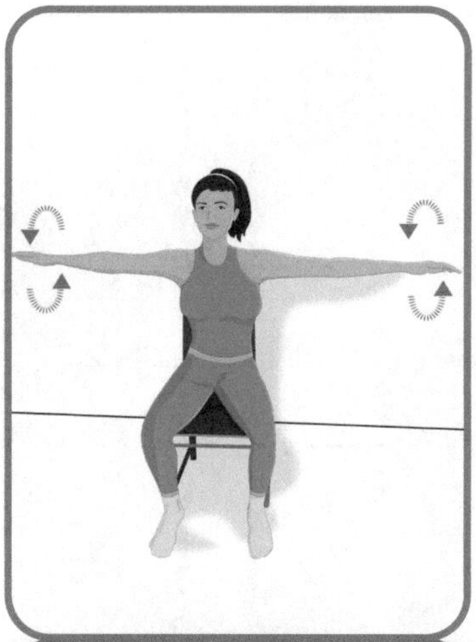

Chair Arm Rotation
Pag 16

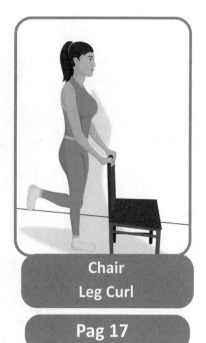

Chair Leg Curl
Pag 17

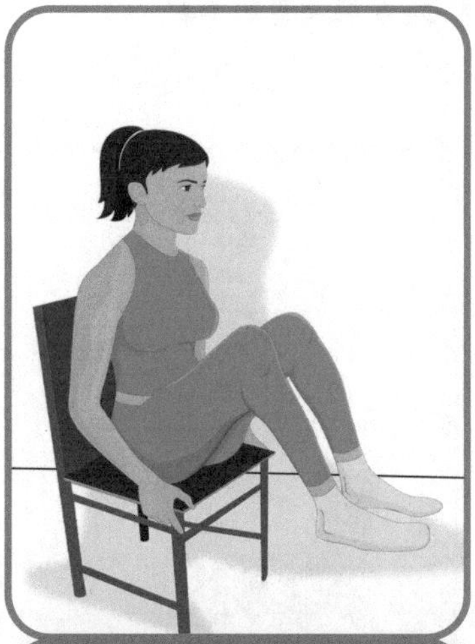

Chair Knee Raise
Pag 18

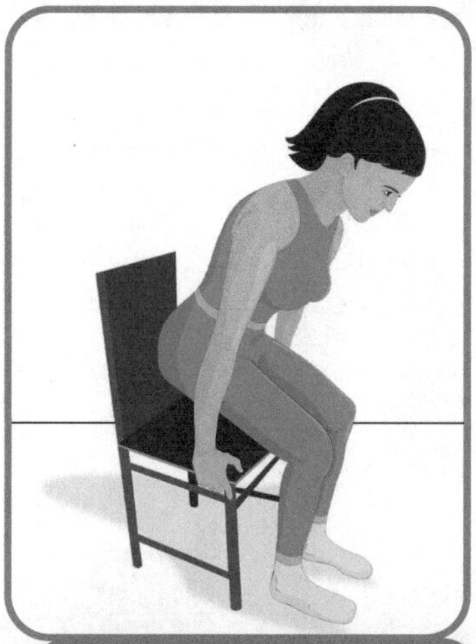

Chair Elevating Hips
Pag 19

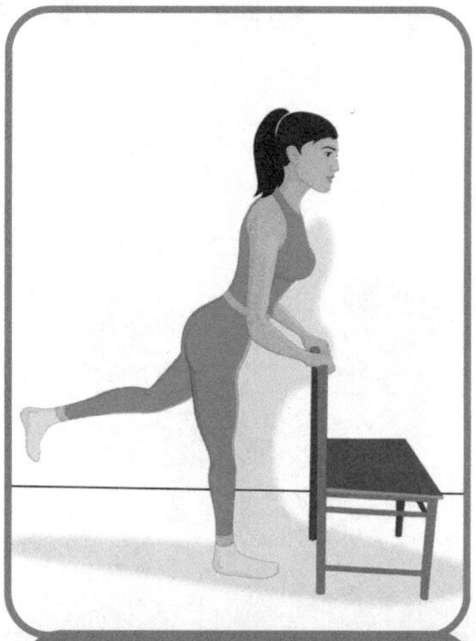

Chair Glute Extension
Pag 20

CHAIR YOGA CARDIO

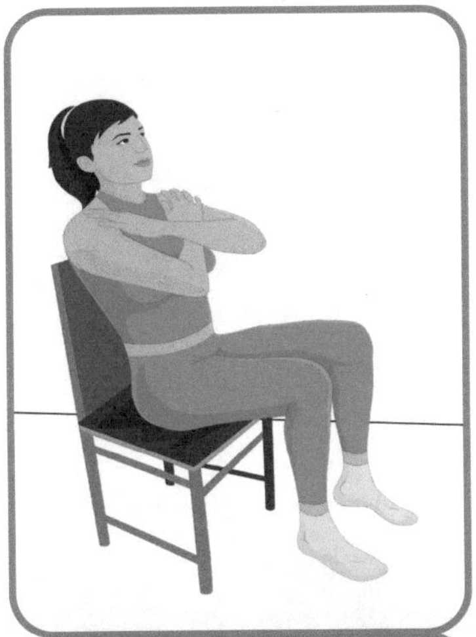

Chair Squat
+ Swing

Pag 21

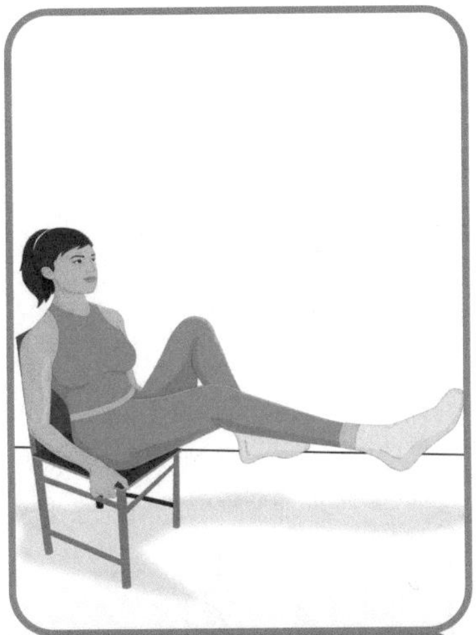

Chair
Cycling

Pag 23

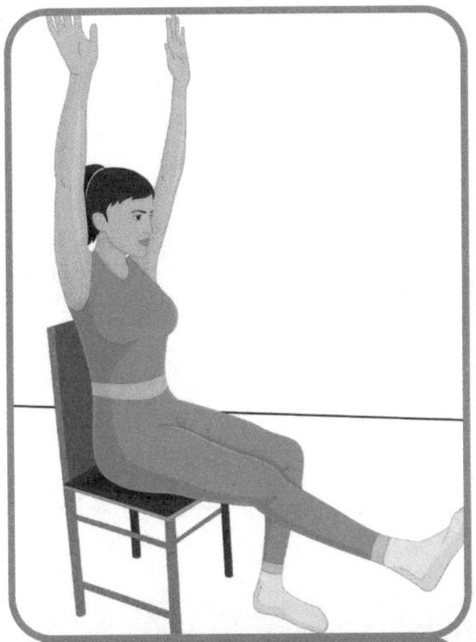

Chair Lifted Arm
+ Leg Kick

Pag 24

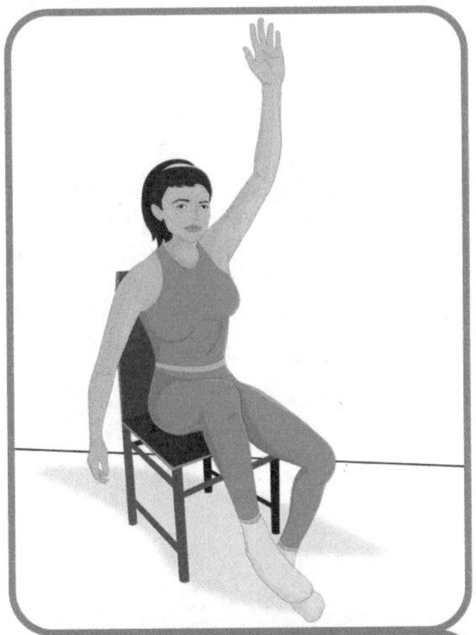

Chair
Full March

Pag 25

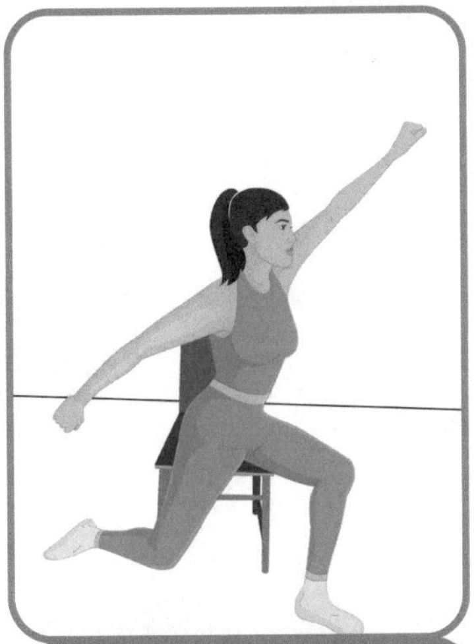

Chair
Superhero Twist

Pag 27

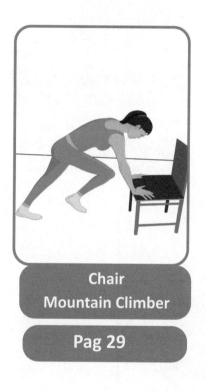

Chair
Mountain Climber

Pag 29

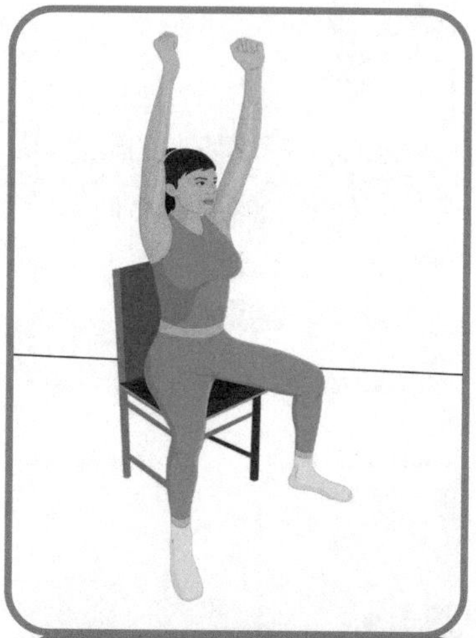

Chair Press
And Open

Pag 30

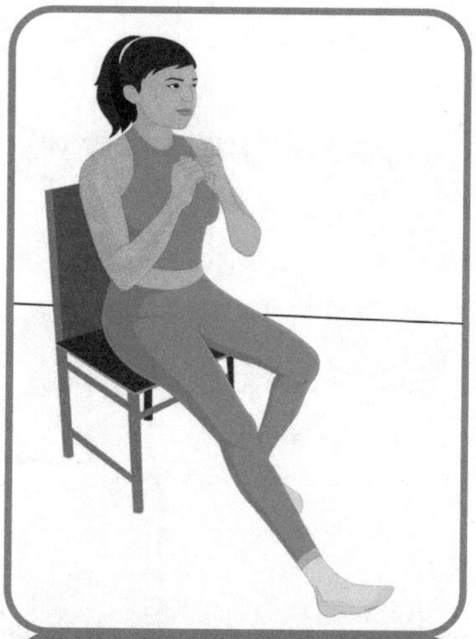

Chair Step + Knee
Touch

Pag 31

ChairYoga

Guess what? Here are gifts for you 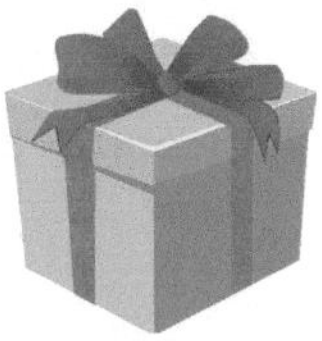

- Special and direct way to text me if you have any questions or just want to say "hi!"
- A simple, easy-to-use printable chart + a personalized follow-up plan to help you stay active and independent

Don't like texting? No problem! Email me anytime at **avfitness99coaching@gmail.com**

I'm here to help you with your fitness!

INTRODUCTION

Chair Yoga is an incredibly beneficial training book that is both challenging and effective, all while using only a chair as your tool. This practice provides excellent results through low-impact exercises, perfect for people aiming to lose weight.

This book will guide you through the process of achieving not only exceptional weight loss (keep in mind that nutrition also plays a role) but also you'll notice more strength and a better fitness level. The structured workout programs have been thoughtfully designed, with the promise that if you commit to them for 28 days, you will notice significant improvements that will positively change your daily life.

I do think that Chair Yoga is about more than just improving your physical fitness; it's about embracing a healthier, more vibrant way of life.

These are the main benefits of Chair Yoga:

Low-Impact and Great Results

Chair Yoga is a game-changer! Unlike many other practices that are known to be very hard on the body to deliver great results in weight loss, Chair Yoga is unique in its own way as it`s gentle yet highly effective, delivering amazing results. The best part is, that the more effort you invest, the more you gain. Chair Yoga carries little risk of injury or overtraining while offering numerous exercise benefits. But here's the real magic: it enhances your overall well-being with a variety of complex advantages.

Burn Calories and Lose Weight

The common belief that sitting for extended periods of time is harmful to your health holds true, but Chair Yoga brings a paradigm change. Whether you work a traditional 9-to-5 office job, work from home, or lead an active lifestyle, the diverse workouts in this book provide a unique and effective way to burn calories and lose weight. Engaging in these exercises on a regular basis will help you increase the amount of calories you burn, and the real results will begin to show when you remain in a consistent routine.

Improved Strength

These exercises boost strength and overall body harmony with a focus on full-body training, leading to strength gains. Even better, most workouts use just bodyweight, so no extra equipment is needed. All you need is willpower, a chair, and 15 minutes!

Improved Flexibility

The majority of the exercises in this book encourage stretching and activation of previously unnoticed body parts, revitalizing and energizing your entire body. Improved flexibility not only improves fitness but also your daily life. The transformations you'll go through will be truly amazing, leaving you feeling younger, more alive, and energized than ever before!

Increased Sense of Peace and Reduced Stress

This form of exercise is really beneficial for developing inner calm and managing stress more effectively. Take your time during the training without other distractions. This will increase the workout's effectiveness and foster a greater sense of calm and well-being by connecting more deeply with your body, emotions, and surroundings.

Improved Posture

In addition to poor breathing, sedentary habits, and a lack of fitness, poor posture is a common issue among many people. The exercises included here will help improve your posture by opening up your body and strengthening underused muscles, such as your back and core muscles. You can expect not only weight loss results but also a significant improvement in your posture within 28 days, provided you stay consistent, of course.

HOW TO READ THE BOOK FOR BEST RESULTS

This book is structured in two main parts: the former shows you the exercises, while the latter explains to you the 28-day plan.

In the first part, every exercise is explained thoroughly with a description that tells you how to perform the movement clearly and effectively.

On top of that, the provided illustrations help you to understand and master the execution. The exercises are numerous and they are divided into 3 sections: Chair Yoga Stretches, Chair Yoga Strengthening, and Chair Yoga Cardio. Also, in the explanation of the exercises, it will not be stated the amount of reps you have to perform on each exercise. This is because the 28-day plan mentioned it.

Note: if you have any questions or doubts regarding the execution of the exercises or any other doubts training related, feel free to email me at **chairyogafreecall@gmail.com**

In the second part, you will see the chapter called "28-Day Plan". You will become very familiar with it as it outlines the exercises to do daily and how many times to perform each one. It is a 28-day plan, every day is being analyzed and prepared to provide you with the best results. Therefore if you want to be successful, reach your goals, and lose weight with low-impact exercise, it is necessary to follow the plan, don't skip days, and enjoy the process.

Enjoy the book! Good luck!

CHAIR YOGA STRETCHES

CHAIR TWIST

This exercise is useful to keep your spine mobile and flexible.

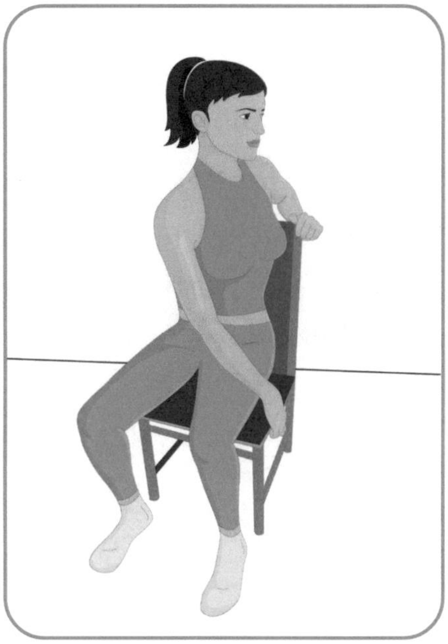

How to Do it:

1. Sit comfortably on a chair with your back straight. From there rotate your back towards the left side. Place your right hand on the left side of the chair. Place your left hand on the chair backrest, as shown.
2. Hold that position for 2 seconds whilst breathing fully - exhale longer than inhale.
3. Then, come back into the starting position and repeat on the other side.
4. Repeat for the total mentioned reps.

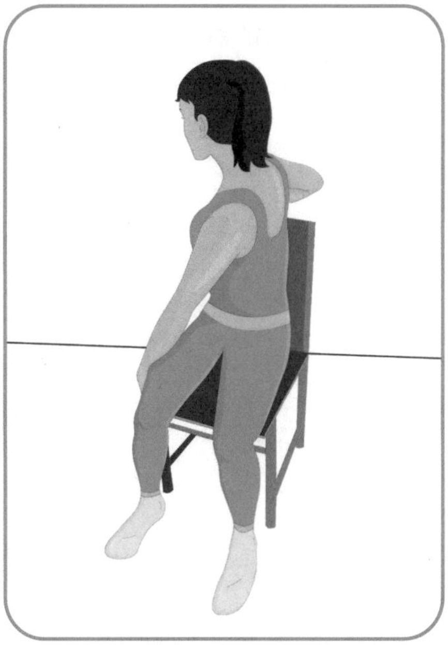

Note:

Make sure not to tense your shoulder or upper back but try your best to keep your muscles relaxed. This will help the effectiveness of the exercise.

CHAIR SIDE OPENING

Great exercise to work on your obliques, helping with toning and stretching the side of your abs.

How to Do it:

1. Sit with your legs wide open, your left arm on your stomach, and your right arm straight over your head.
2. From there, bend your back towards the left side as much as you feel comfortable. Exhale as you do so.
3. Hold the position for 1 second, then come back into the starting position, and repeat on the other side.

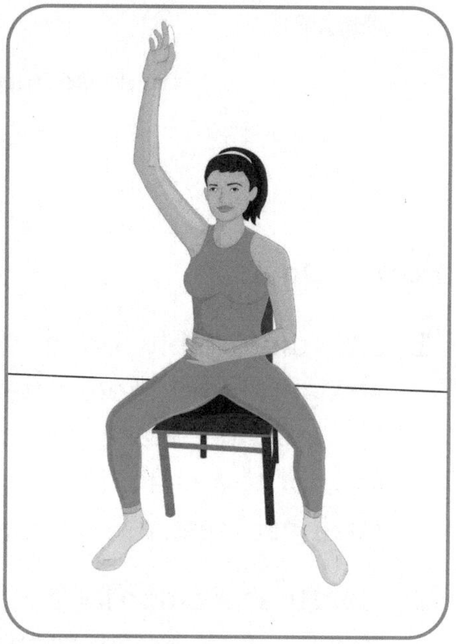

Note:

Initially, limited motion is normal. With practice, you'll gain flexibility and notice stronger, leaner side abs.

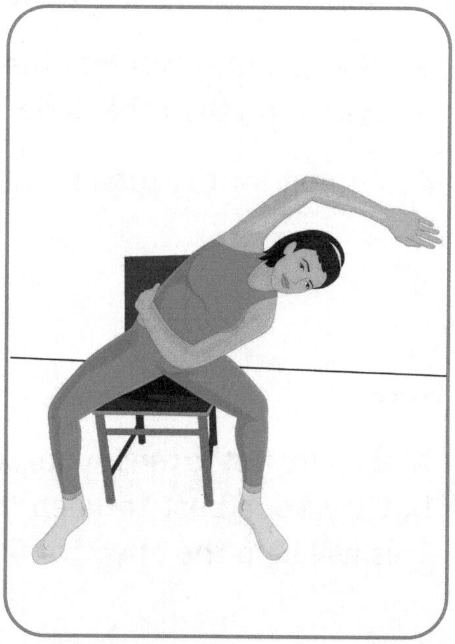

CHAIR BACK STRETCH

This exercise is excellent for spine stretching, improving posture, and preventing injuries and back issues.

How to Do it:

1. Stand in front of a chair approximately two to three feet away from it, depending on your height.
2. Place your hands on the backrest, and lean forward by bending at your hips. Your back will be stretched.
3. Hold the position for the mentioned seconds.

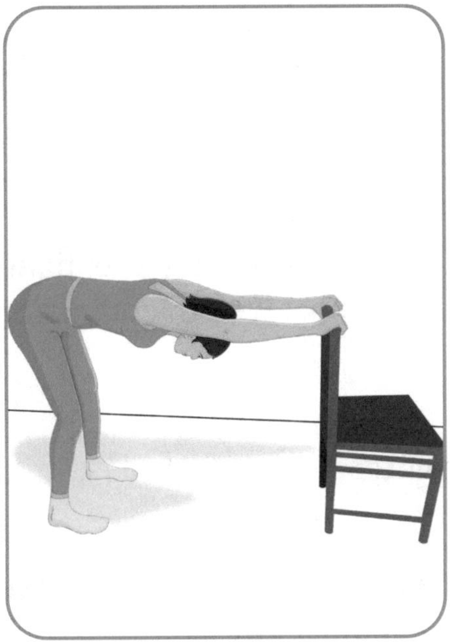

Note:

Feel free to slightly bend your knees as you keep the position. This will put less stretch on the back of your legs, focusing more on stretching your back.

CHAIR TRICEPS STRETCH

A simple stretch for your arms. It's simple and effective...Try to believe it!

How to Do it:

1. Sit comfortably on a chair, and bring your left arm over your head - Bend your elbow as you do so.
2. Next, use your right arm to gently push your left elbow to the right, and you'll begin to feel the stretch on the back of the left arm.
3. Remember to keep breathing as you perform this movement.
4. Hold it for the mentioned seconds, and then repeat with the other arm.

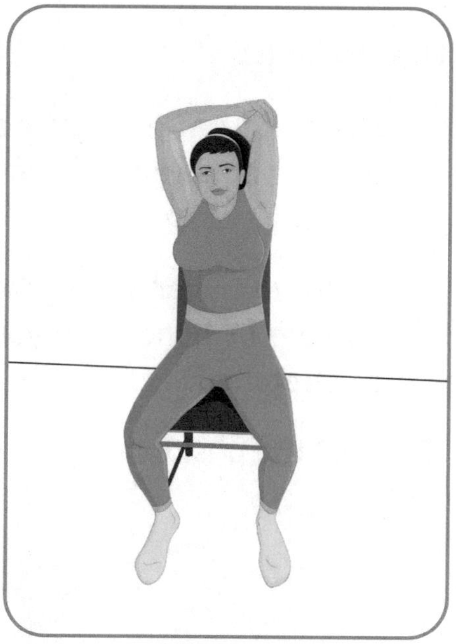

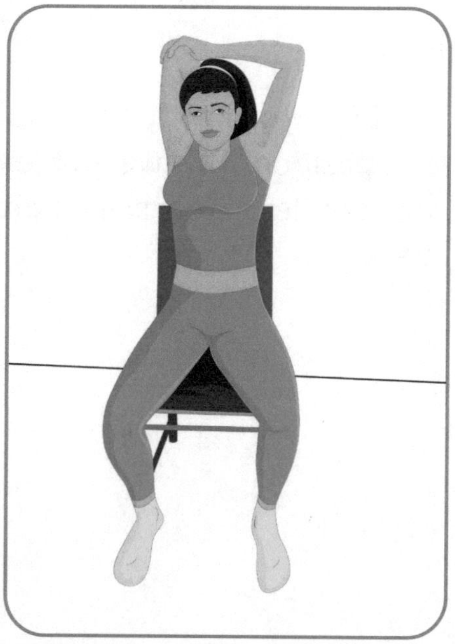

Note:

Keep your neck and shoulders relaxed. There may be times when you instinctively lift them. Be mindful of this.

CHAIR GLUTE STRETCH

A fantastic exercise to stretch your glutes and the outside of your thighs. Great for enhancing hip mobility too.

How to Do it:

1. Sit comfortably on a chair, Place your left ankle on your right thigh. Push gently your left knee towards the floor with your left hand.
2. Hold the stretch for the mentioned seconds.
3. Then, repeat on the other side.

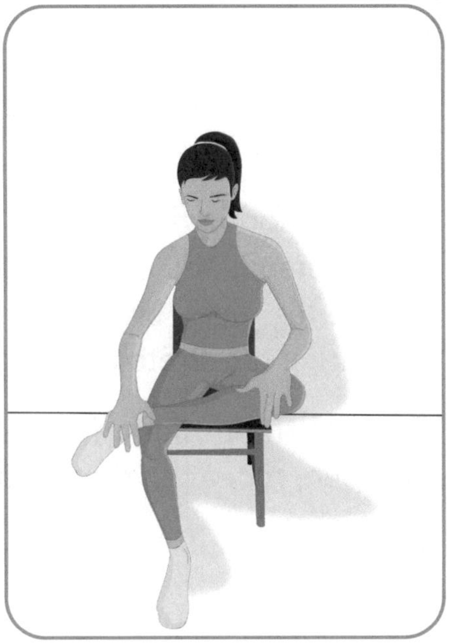

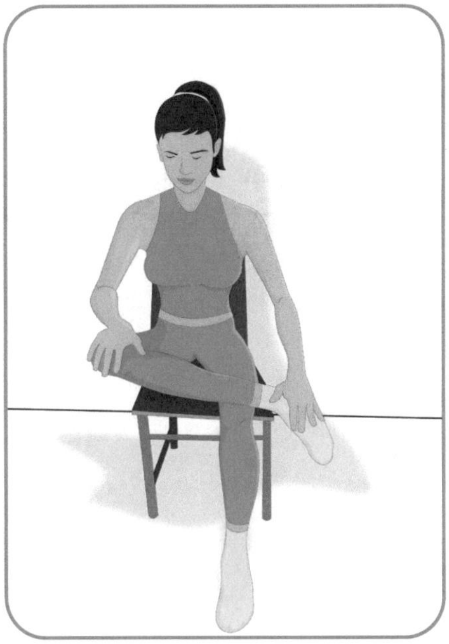

Note:

Ensure you maintain an upright posture to optimize the effectiveness of the glute stretch.

CHAIR CALF STRETCH

A great exercise to stretch the back of your lower leg, one side at a time.

How to Do it:

1. Sit on the brink of the chair and extend your left leg.
2. Lean forward to touch your toes with your left hand. You'll feel a stretch on the back of the leg. Keep breathing slowly and controlled during the stretch.
3. Hold the position for the mentioned seconds. Then, repeat on the other side.

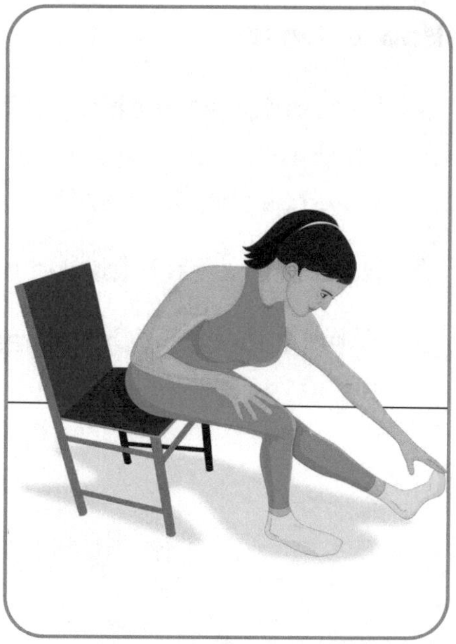

Note:

A slight knee bend is acceptable, but for a deeper stretch, aim to keep it straight whenever possible.

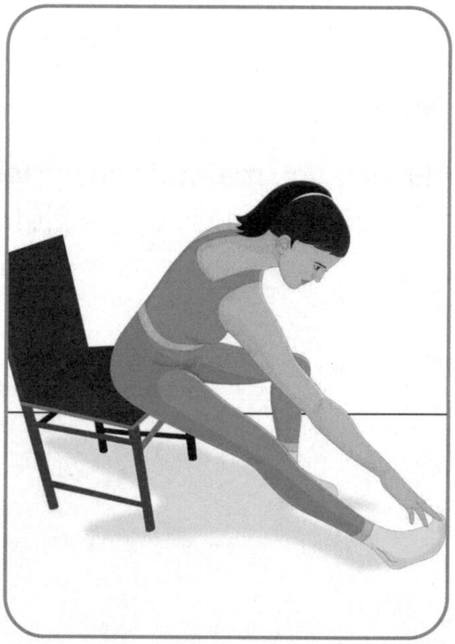

CHAIR OPENING CHEST

Great stretch for opening up your chest and releasing some tension on your upper body.

How to Do it:

1. Sit leaving some space between your back and the backrest. Place your hands on a chair behind your back.
2. From there, open up your chest and lift your chin. Focus on the stretch on the side of your chest.
3. Hold the position for the mentioned seconds.

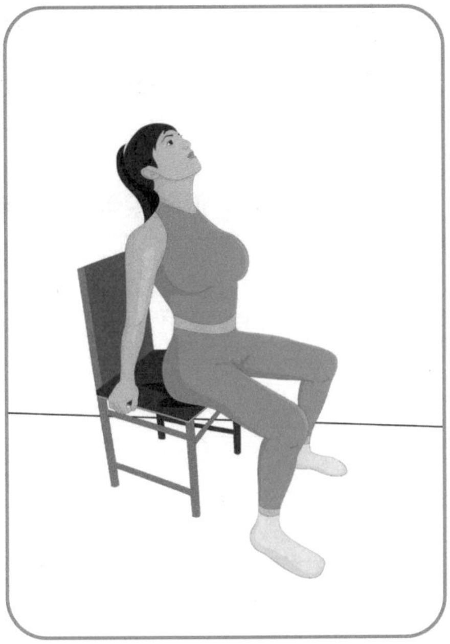

Note:

This stretch is highly effective for quickly relieving upper body tension. Ensure you keep breathing throughout and avoid holding your breath.

CHAIR FORWARD FOLD

This exercise is excellent for stretching your lower back and reducing tension in that area.

How to Do it:

1. Sit comfortably with your feet shoulder-width apart, and your arms on the side, as shown.
2. Slowly fold your back forward until your chest touches your thighs, Keep your chin tucked.
3. Then, slowly come back up into the starting position.
4. Repeat for the specified number of reps.

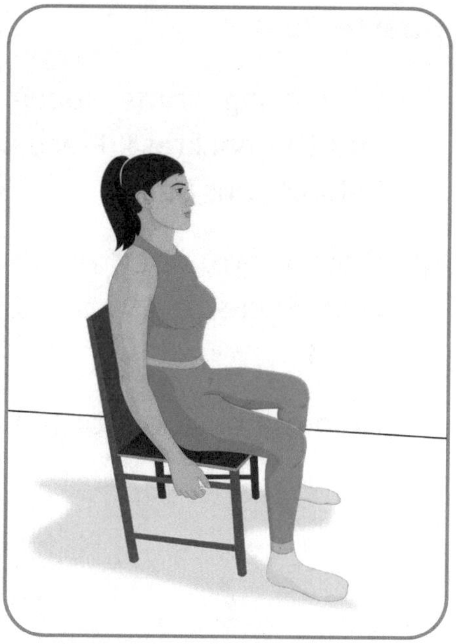

Note:

I recommend performing this exercise slowly and with control, particularly if you're new to it. Moving too quickly can be more harmful than beneficial.

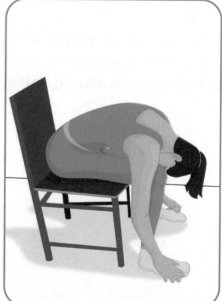

CHAIR YOGA STRENGTHENING

CHAIR PUSH UP

A simple yet very effective exercise for strengthening your arms, shoulders, and chest as well as improving your body awareness.

How to Do it:

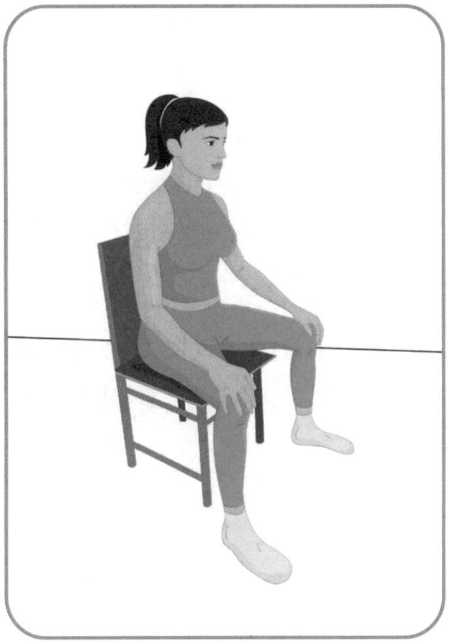

1. Sit on a chair with feet slightly wider than shoulder width apart and hands on your thighs. Keep your back straight.
2. From there, lean forward by bending at your hips until your chest is almost touching your thighs.
3. Exhale as you come back into the starting position, and repeat for the specified number of reps.

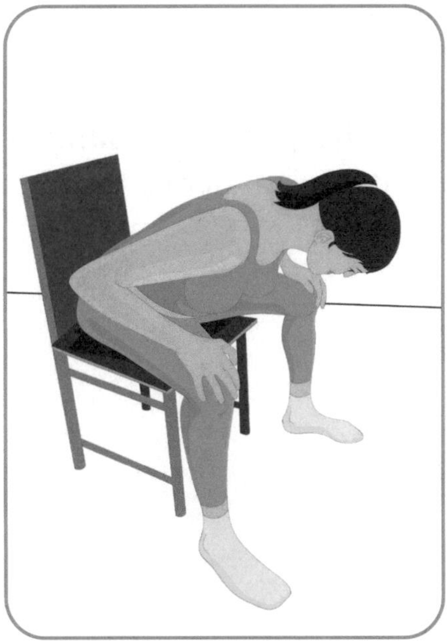

Note:

This is a simplified version of push-ups. If you find it challenging, limit your range of motion to a comfortable yet still challenging level. Make sure not to tense your trunk as it would make the exercise more difficult to execute. A controlled and constant breath, rather than holding it, would help prevent doing so.

CHAIR CALF RAISES

A great exercise to strengthen your feet, ankles, and calves muscles.

How to Do it:

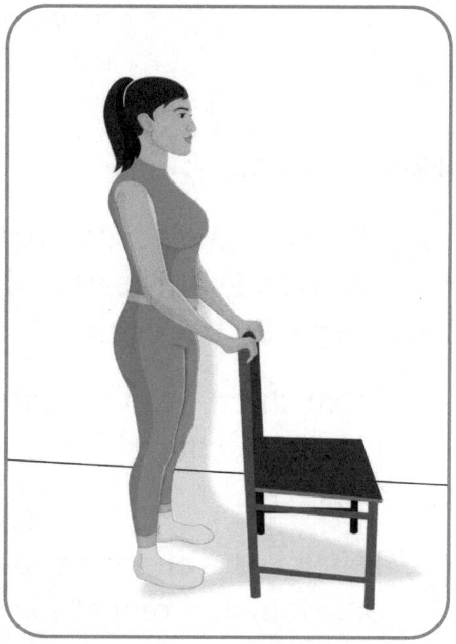

1. Stand in front of a chair's backrest with your hands on it. Feet slightly closer than shoulder width apart.
2. Lift your heels as high as you can whilst keeping your body straight. Hold that position for one second.
3. Then, return to the starting position, and repeat for the specified number of reps.

Note:

To increase the challenge, use less support from the chair, allowing your feet to bear more of your body weight during the exercise.

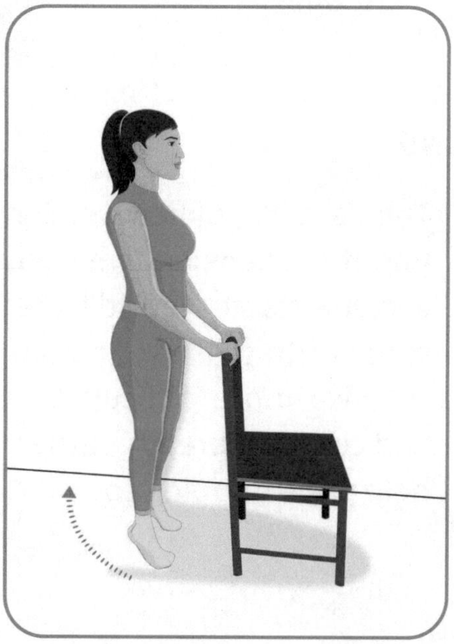

CHAIR SQUAT

Great compound exercise that targets all your leg muscles as well as increasing your heart rate.

How to Do it:

1. Sit comfortably on a chair with feet shoulder-width apart, back straight, and hands on the opposite shoulder as shown in the images.
2. From there, lift yourself up pushing your feet against the floor.
3. Then, come back into the starting position, and repeat for the mentioned reps.

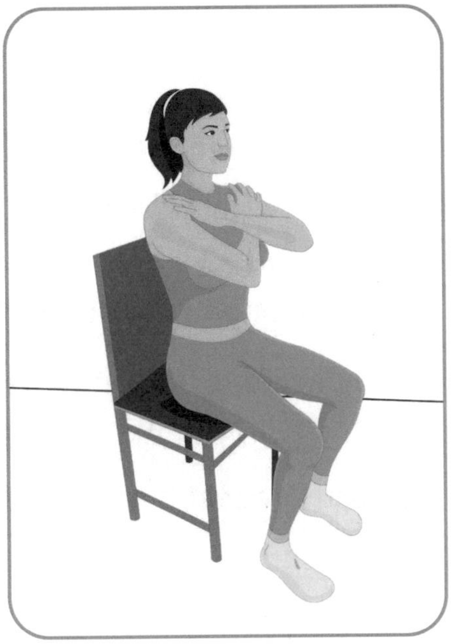

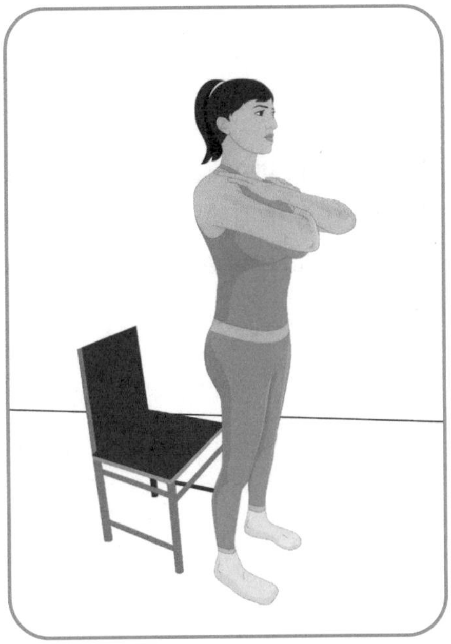

Note:

If you find this exercise too challenging, you can place your hands on the chair to assist yourself when getting up.

CHAIR LEG EXTENSION

This exercise aims to strengthen the quadriceps and maintain healthy knees.

How to Do it:

1. Sit comfortably on a chair with your back straight. Hands holding the side of the chair as shown in the first image.
2. Straight one leg while keeping both thighs on the chair and the opposite foot on the floor.
3. Then, come back into the starting position and repeat it for the mentioned reps.
4. Lastly, repeat it on the other side.

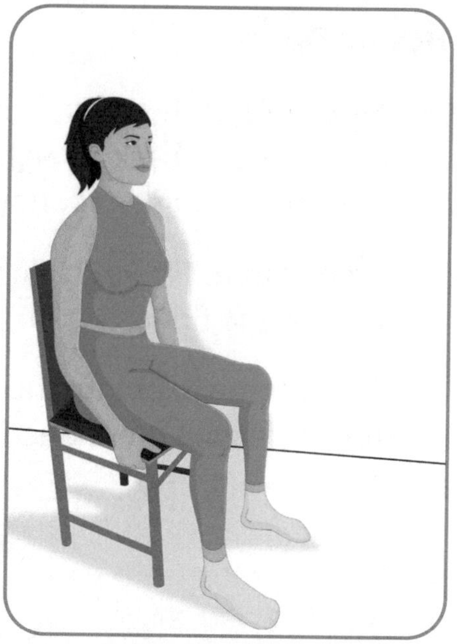

Note:

Lift your leg faster on the way up than when lowering it down. If it's too easy, using an ankle weight can be a good idea (not necessary, though).

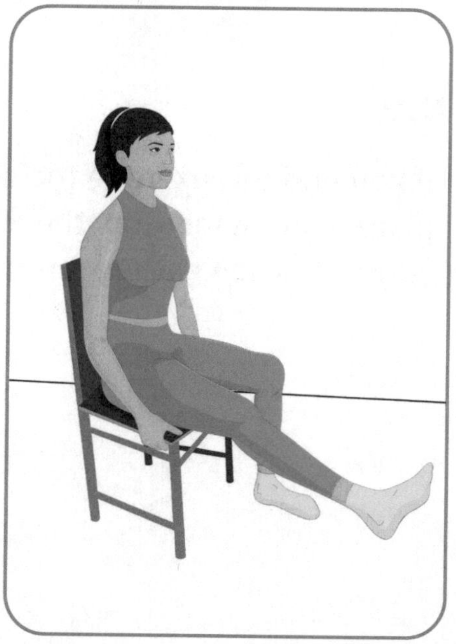

CHAIR ARM ROTATION

Chair arm rotation is a wonderful exercise that strengthens the arms and shoulders.

How to Do it:

1. Assume a comfortable seated position in a chair, ensuring your spine is upright and aligned. Next, extend your arms out to the sides, as though you're forming a cross.
2. Rotate both arms in a clockwise motion, creating hand-drawn circles.
3. Repeat for the specified number of reps and then repeat it in the counterclockwise direction.

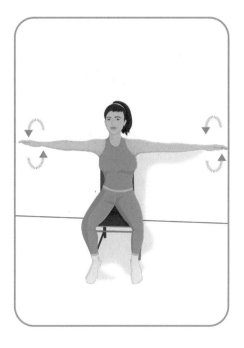

Note:

To make it more difficult, move slowly as it requires you to work on your arms for an extended duration. Therefore, it's advisable not to rush the movement to fully reap its benefits.

CHAIR LEG CURL

This exercise is designed to improve balance, strengthen the hamstrings, and keep your knees healthy.

How to Do it:

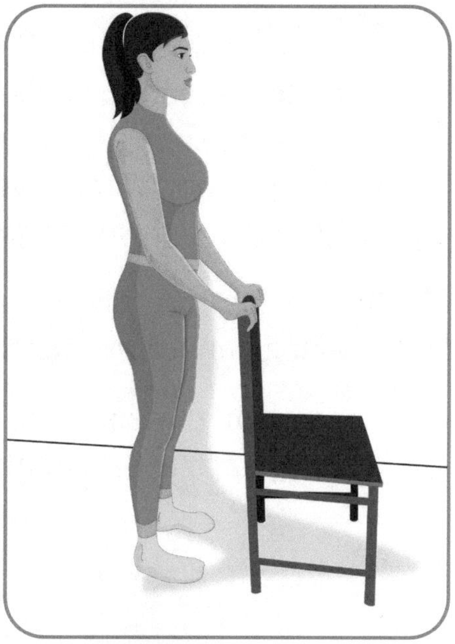

1. Stand straight while holding onto a chair`s backrest in front of you.
2. Lift your heel and hold that position for 1 second whilst breathing fully - exhale longer than inhale.
3. Then, come back into the starting position and repeat for the specified number of reps.
4. Lastly, repeat it on the other side.

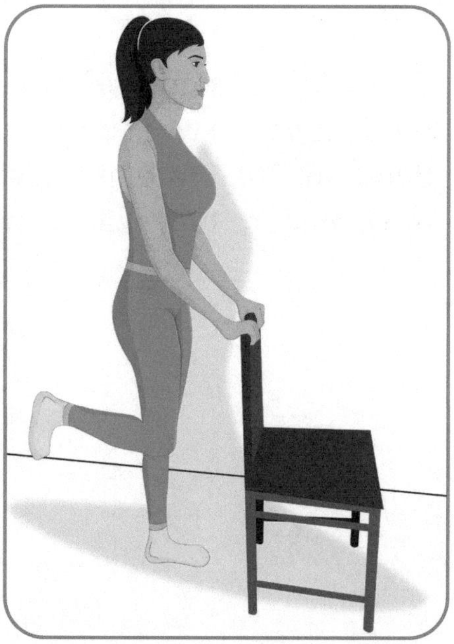

Note:

Make sure not to tense your shoulder or upper back but try your best to keep your muscles relaxed. It is a relatively easy exercise that can be done successfully by beginners too.

To make it more difficult, increase the range of motion aiming to touch your glute with your heel.

CHAIR KNEE RAISE

Wonderful exercise to strengthen your core and improve your flexibility.

How to Do it:

1. Sit comfortably on a chair with your back straight. Hands holding the side of the chair.
2. Raise both your knees while engaging your core, maintaining an upright spine, and gripping the sides of the chair with your hands.
3. Then, come back into the starting position and repeat the movement for the mentioned reps.

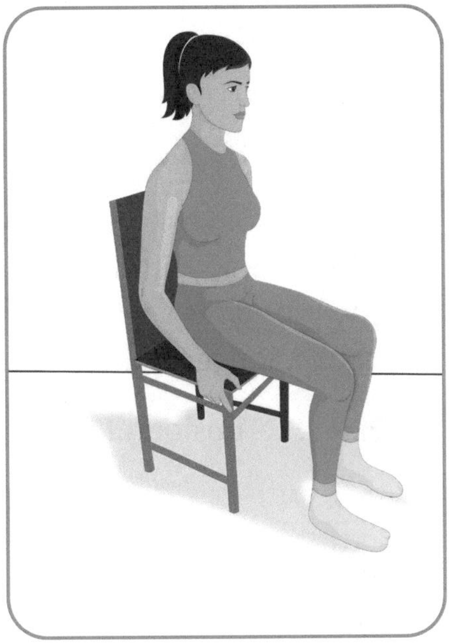

Note:

Keep in mind to inhale as you lift your knees and exhale as you lower them. The slower you perform the lowering phase, the more challenging it becomes.

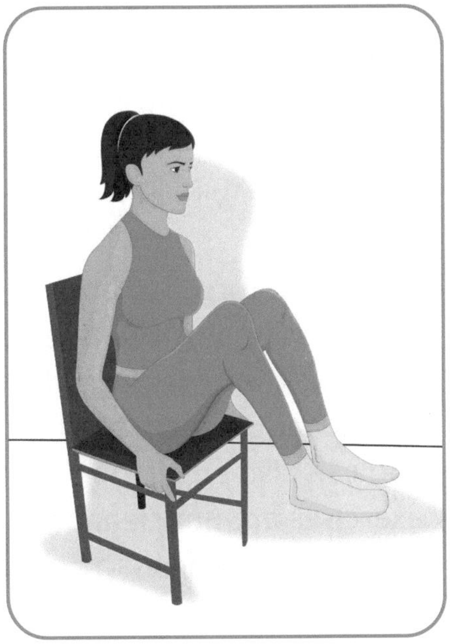

CHAIR ELEVATING HIPS

This exercise is great to strengthen your arms and core.

How to Do it:

1. Sit comfortably on a chair with your back straight. Hands holding the side of the chair.
2. Extend your arms fully, and your glutes and hips will naturally lift as well. Hold that position for the mentioned seconds whilst breathing fully - exhale longer than inhale.
3. Hold the position for the mentioned seconds.

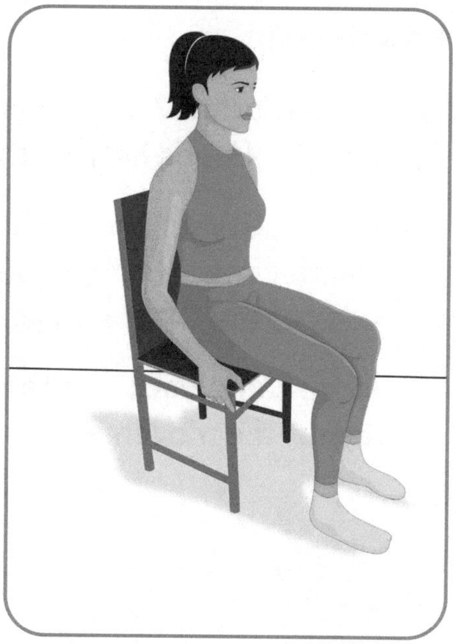

Note:
While it may appear simple, holding this position can be quite challenging, especially for beginners. Concentrate on your breathing to make it more manageable. You'll notice your arms and shoulders doing the majority of the work, along with engaging your core.

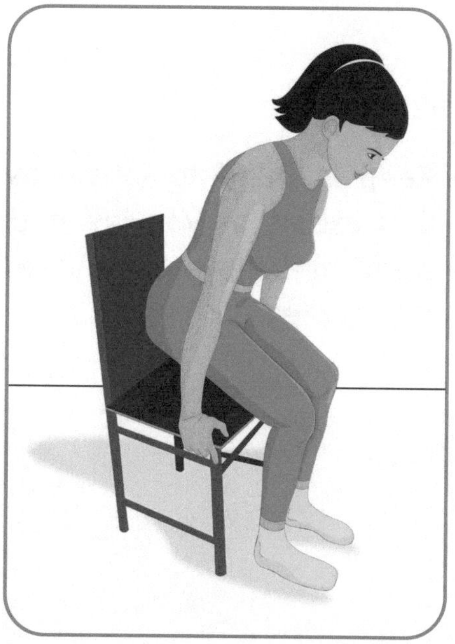

Hey, don't forget to book your free 1-on-1 Chair Yoga session in a video call with me. Write "FREE CALL" at **chairyogafreecall@gmail.com** and let's schedule the training.
You can also email me anytime you need if some exercises are not clear or you have some doubts about something in the book!

CHAIR GLUTE EXTENSION

This exercise is perfect for toning and strengthening your glutes.

How to Do it:

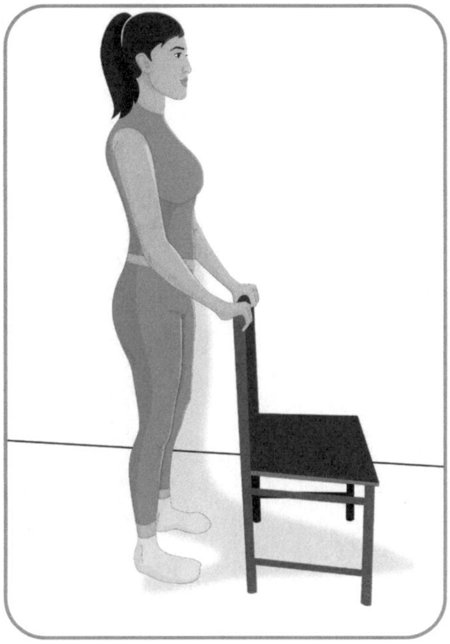

1. Stand straight while holding onto a chair`s backrest in front of you.
2. Then, extend your left leg behind you and hold that position for 2 seconds. Breath fully - exhale as you extend the leg.
3. Then, come back into the starting position and repeat for the mentioned reps.
4. Lastly, perform the movement with the other side.

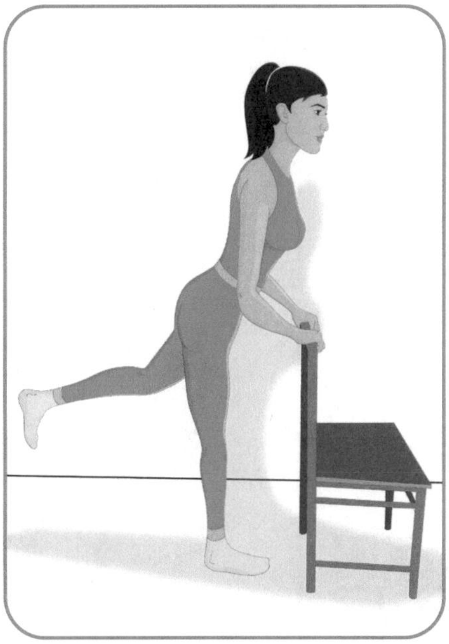

Note:

Be mindful not to tense your shoulders or upper back; aim to keep these muscles relaxed. Instead, focus on activating your glutes when lifting your leg, as this maximizes the benefits of the exercise.

CHAIR YOGA CARDIO

CHAIR SQUAT + SWING

It strengthens your legs while increasing your heart rate and general fitness with a fun and dynamic exercise.

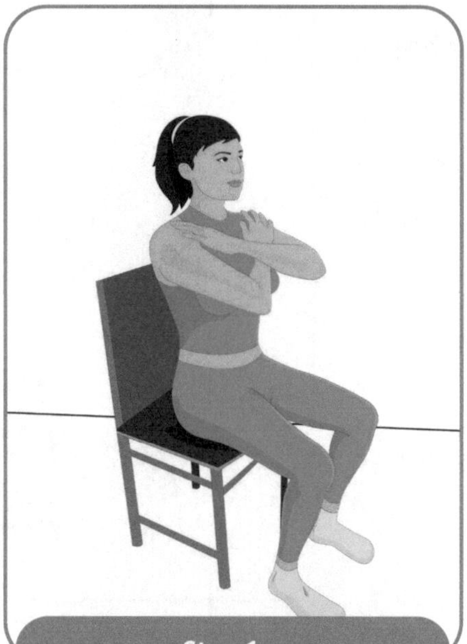

Step 1

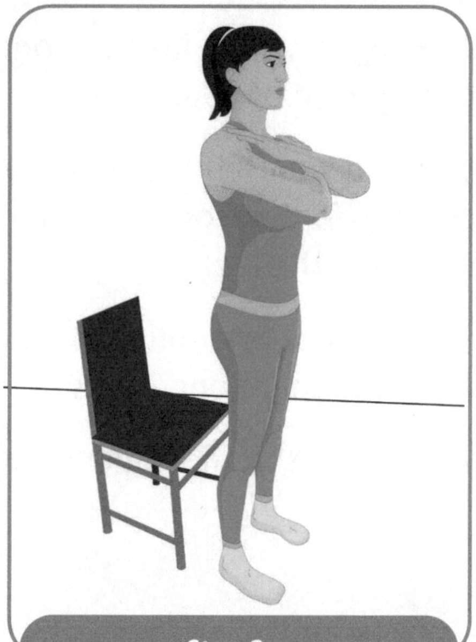

Step 2

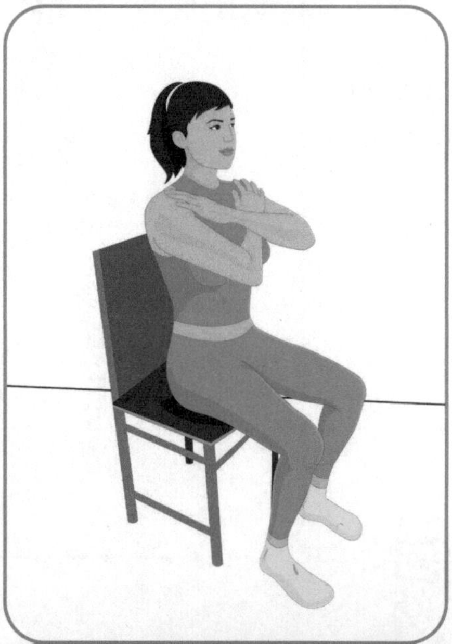

Step 3

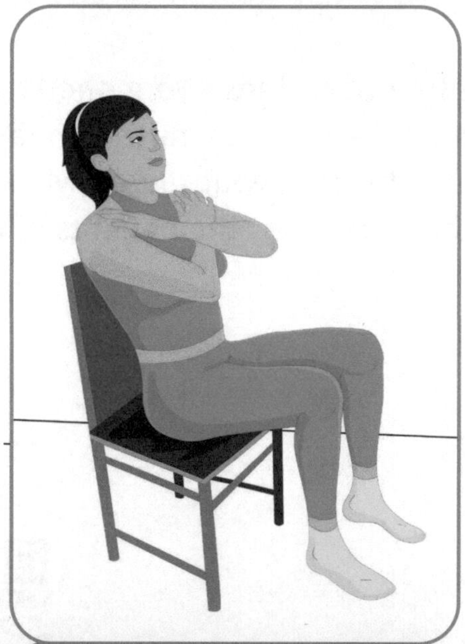

Step 4

How to Do it:

1. Sit on a chair with your back straight, your feet slightly wider than shoulder-width apart and your hands on the opposite shoulder with your arms crossed and parallel to the floor, as shown in the image.
2. From there, lift yourself by using your legs.
3. Then, return to the initial position. When you sit, raise your knees, and use the momentum to stand again as soon as your feet touch the floor.
4. Repeat for the mentioned reps.

Note:

This exercise is one of the most dynamic here. No worries if you feel tired after just a few reps; that's completely normal (actually, it's good for your progress!)

CHAIR CYCLING

This is an excellent exercise that not only helps you burn calories but also gently tones your abs.

How to Do it:

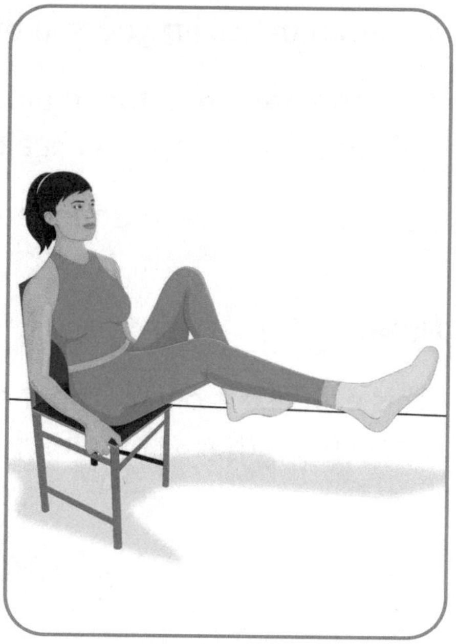

1. Sit on the brink of the chair with your hands holding on it as shown. Lift your legs and have one leg almost straight and the other one with the knee bent. Make sure to have both legs in the air as the first image shows.
2. From there, simply "cycle through" so that the straight leg becomes bent, and vice versa.
3. Repeat for the mentioned seconds.

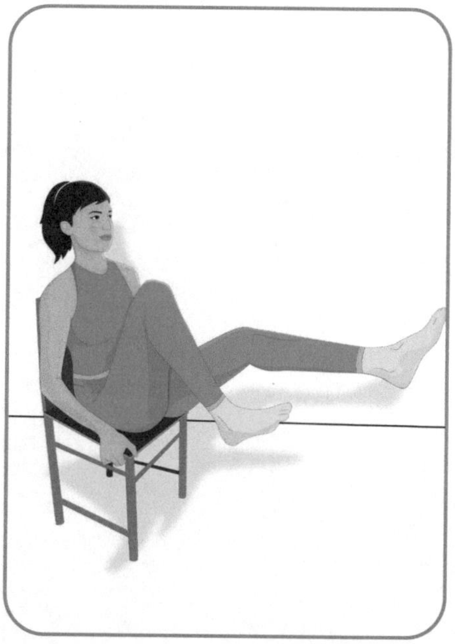

Note:

I'd recommend leaning slightly backward with your torso to enhance your balance and engage your abs more effectively.

if you have any questions or doubts regarding the execution of this exercise (or others) or any other doubts training related, feel free to email me at chairyogafreecall@gmail.com

CHAIR LIFTED ARM +LEG KICK

Fantastic exercises that mix flexibility and weight loss in a simple movement.

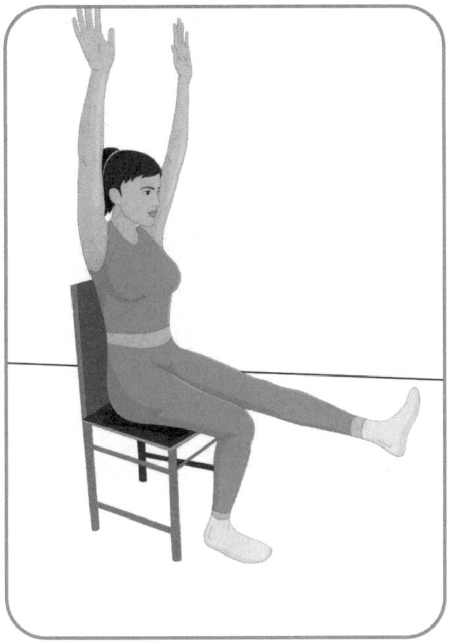

How to Do it:

1. Sit on a chair with your back straight and arms extended overhead. Arms over your head.
2. While maintaining this position, extend the left leg forward.
3. Then, return to the starting position and extend the right leg.
4. Repeat the sequence for the mentioned seconds.

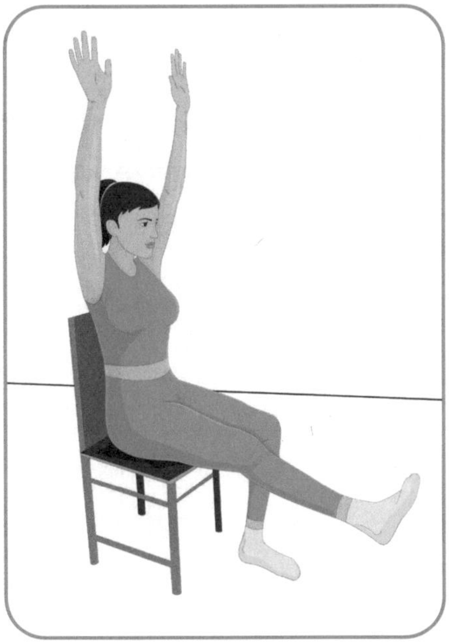

Note:

The faster you move your legs, the more effective it will be for increasing your heart rate, and therefore burning calories.

CHAIR FULL MARCH

An easy and effective full-body exercise to burn calories whilst sitting.

How to Do it:

1. Sit on a chair with your back upright (without leaning onto the chair's backrest) and keep your feet shoulder-width apart.
2. Next, raise your right arm straight overhead along with the left knee.
3. Then, come back to the starting position, and repeat it on the other side - Lifting the left arm and right knee as shown in the second image.
4. Repeat the sequence for the specified amount of seconds.

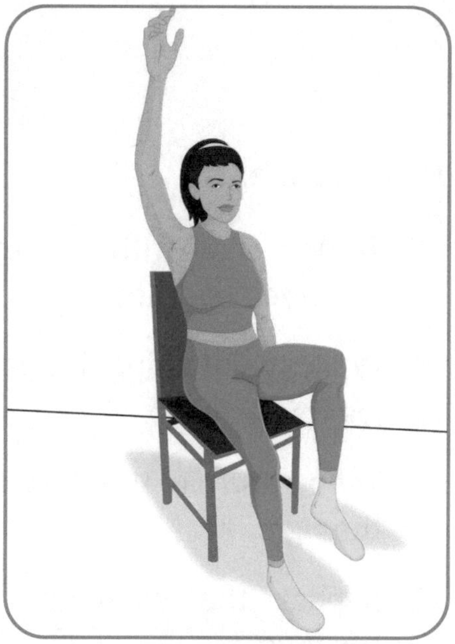

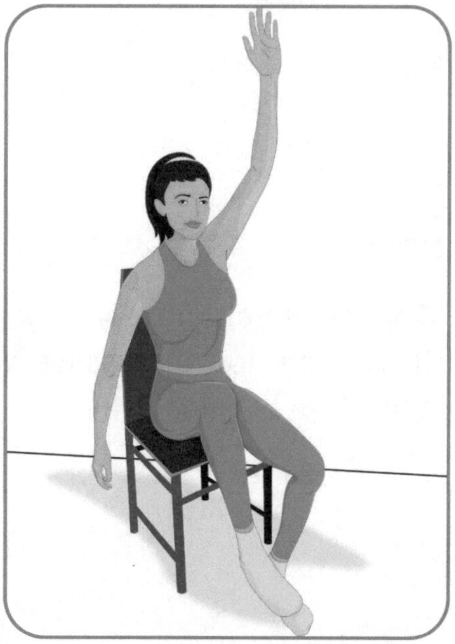

Note:

For your initial attempt, I recommend practicing the movement slowly and with control to get it right. Afterward, try to perform it as quickly as possible to maximize weight loss.

Join Our Community on Facebook for Exclusive Content!

Scan the QR Code Below

CHAIR SUPERHERO TWIST

Cardio exercise that will also improve your hip mobility and coordination.

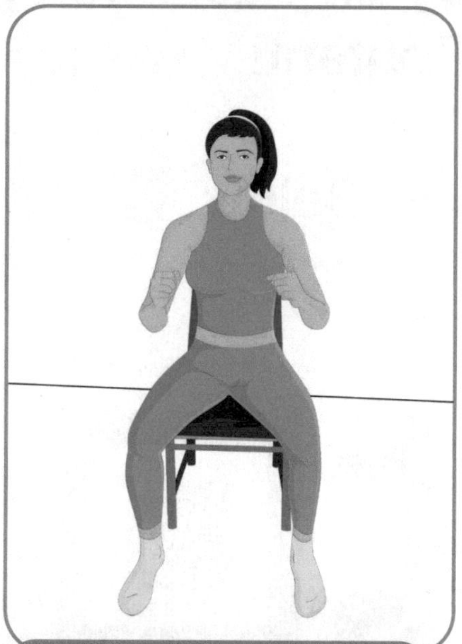

Starting Position

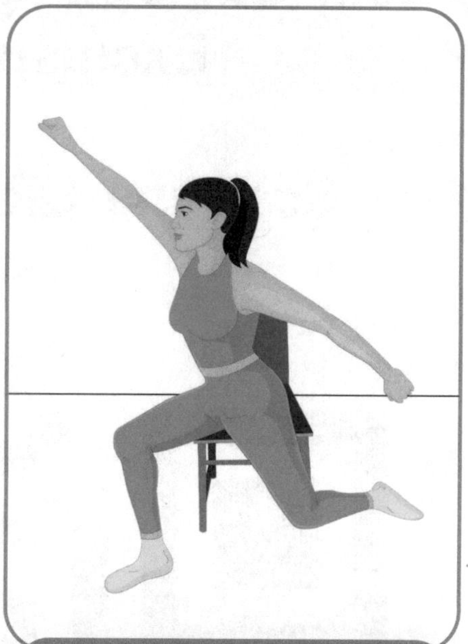

Rotate to the right side

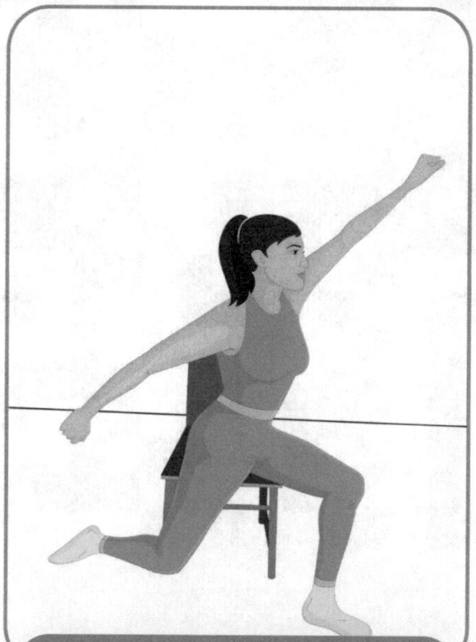

Rotate to the left side

How to Do it:

1. Begin by sitting on a chair with your back upright, your hands positioned in front of your shoulders (with bent elbows), and your feet shoulder-width apart.
2. Next, twist your back in the direction of one side and simultaneously extend the arm on that side, keeping it straight. You can refer to an image for a clearer understanding.
3. Then, come back into the starting position and repeat on the other side.
4. Repeat the whole sequence for the mentioned seconds.

Note:

My suggestion is to initially focus on mastering the technique. Once you've got it down, shift your attention to performing it as quickly as possible.

CHAIR MOUNTAIN CLIMBER

One of the most challenging exercises - great for weight loss, toning your legs and strengthening your abs.

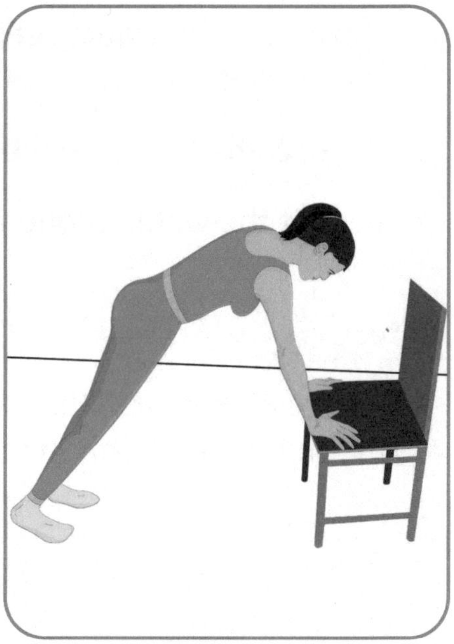

How to Do it:

1. Begin by positioning your hands on the chair and leaning your body forward onto it. Imagine you're in a push-up position with your hands on the chair.
2. From there, lift one knee towards your chest.
3. Then, come back into the starting position and lift the other knee - Try to perform this movement fast.
4. Repeat the sequence for the mentioned seconds.

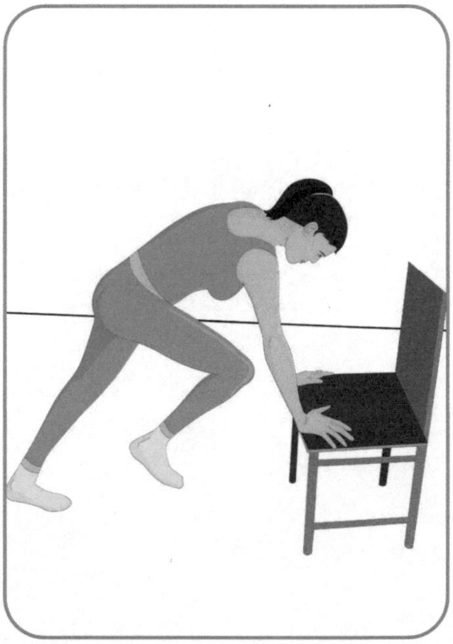

Note:

Ensure you grip the chair firmly with your hands; this way, your arms will also get some exercise.

When you first try it, you can incorporate a brief pause each time you return to the starting position. Over time, the goal is for it to resemble a nearly continuous running-in-place motion.

CHAIR PRESS AND OPEN

This is a straightforward yet effective exercise that integrates both lower and upper body movements, simultaneously enhancing coordination.

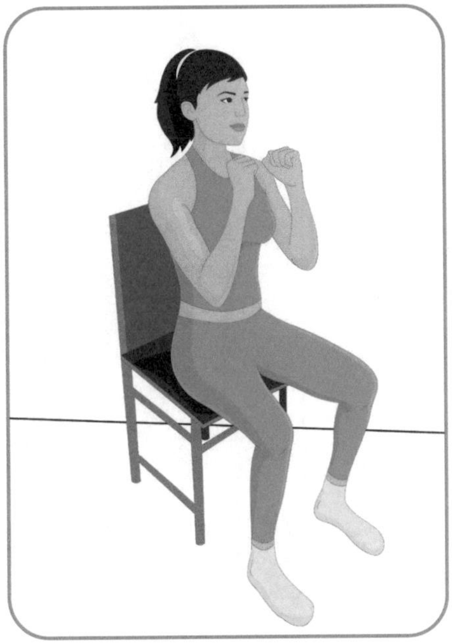

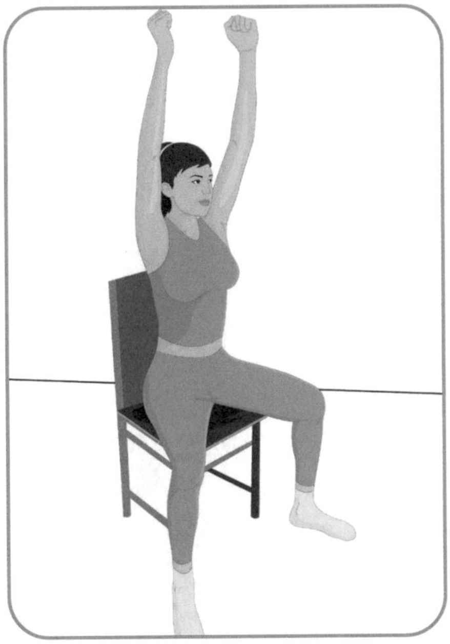

How to Do it:

1. Sit on a chair with your back straight, feet apart, and hands in front of your shoulders, like in the first image.
2. Next, simultaneously widen your legs and raise your fists straight above your head.
3. Come back into the starting position, and repeat for the mentioned reps.

Note:

Start with a limited range of motion, if you currently have limited hip mobility.

Attempting to open your legs too quickly during the exercise could lead to unnecessary hip discomfort.

Instead, if the movement feels too easy, increase the speed of the execution.

CHAIR STEP + KNEE TOUCH

This exercise is an effective combination for working your legs and core, helping to target your stomach and burn extra calories.

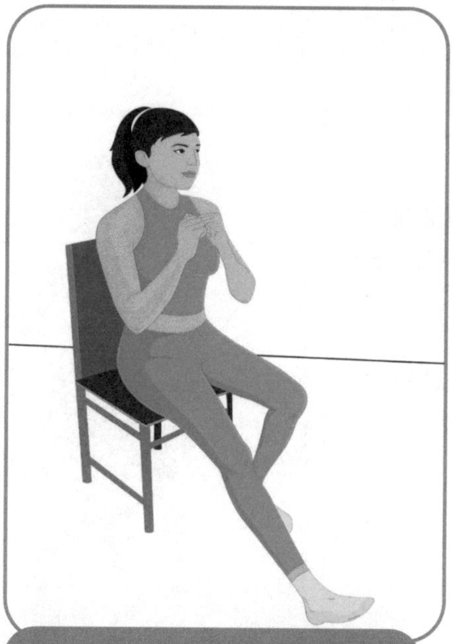

Extend the right foot

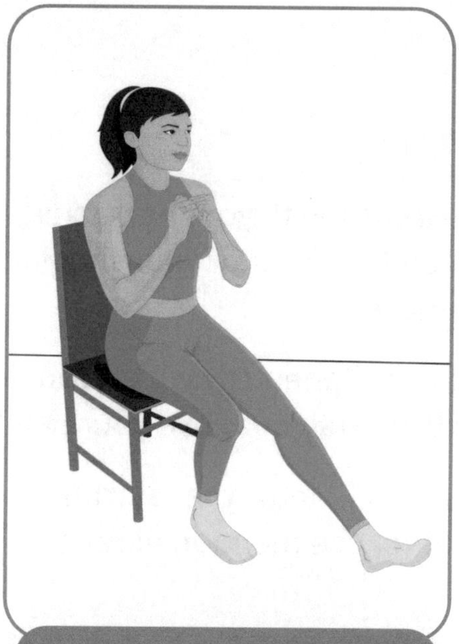

Then, extend the left foot

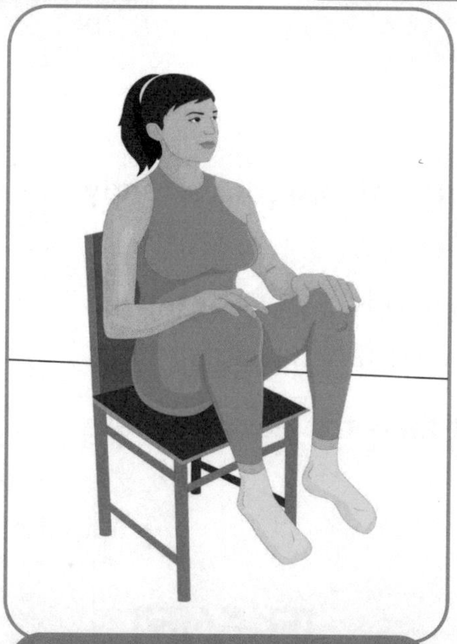

Lastly, raise both legs off the floor

How to Do it:

1. Sit on a chair with your back straight holding your hands in front of your chest.
2. Extend your right leg in front of you while keeping the right heel on the floor.
3. Then, come back into the initial position and repeat on the other side.
4. Finally, return to the starting position and raise both legs off the floor (keeping your knees bent) to touch your knees with your hands.
5. Repeat the whole sequence for the mentioned seconds.

Note:

Great exercise that requires a great combination of coordination, agility, and core strength...I am sure you'll be sweating whilst doing this one! I challenge you to do it faster and faster every time you perform it!

28-DAY PLAN

You can lose weight effectively in just 15-20 minutes of exercise per day with this 28-Day Plan.

The routine here has been proven to strengthen your muscles, make you feel better, and burn calories.

If you can associate those workouts with a healthy diet and enough rest (sleep is crucial for many reasons, including body recomposition. Results will arrive before you know it).

Note: Before each day I'll write "Perform x times'. It means that you will be repeating the whole sequence of the exercise mentioned for that amount of time (Once you finish the last exercise feel free to take 5-10 seconds rest before restarting again with the sequence).

HOW TO READ THE 28 DAY

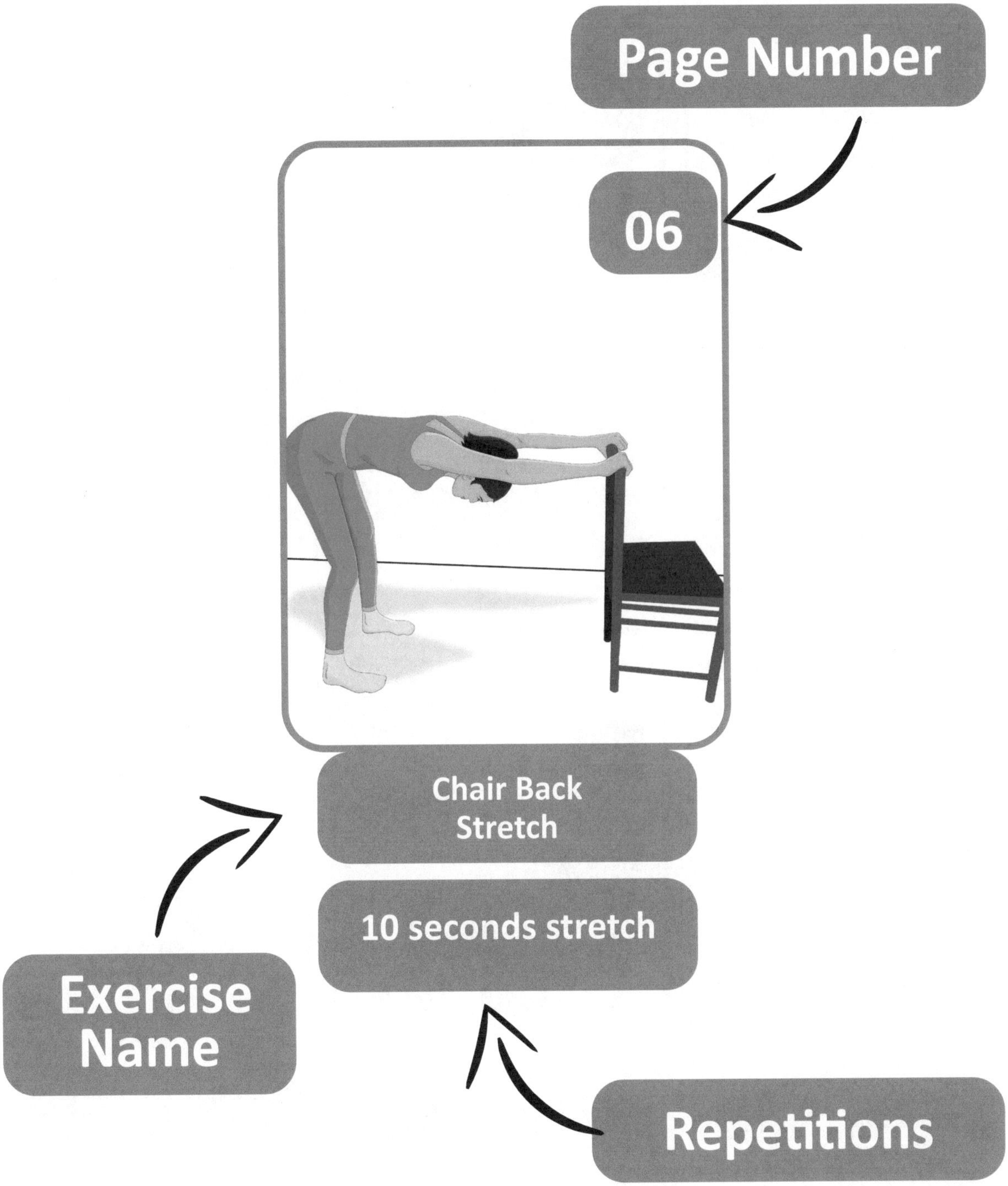

DAY 1 – Perform one to two sets. (The order of the exercises goes from top left to top right, then bottom left to bottom right)

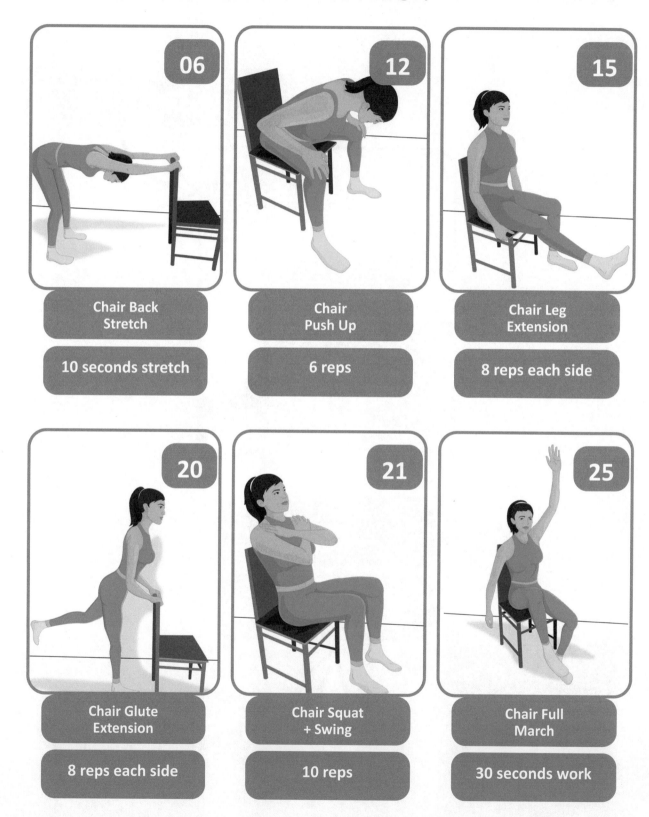

Chair Back Stretch

10 seconds stretch

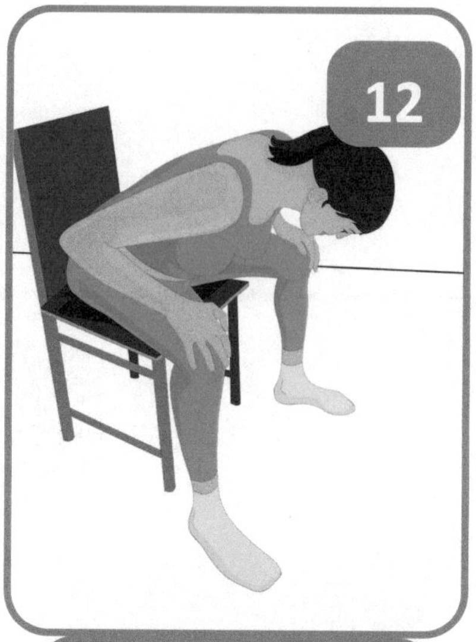

Chair Push Up

6 reps

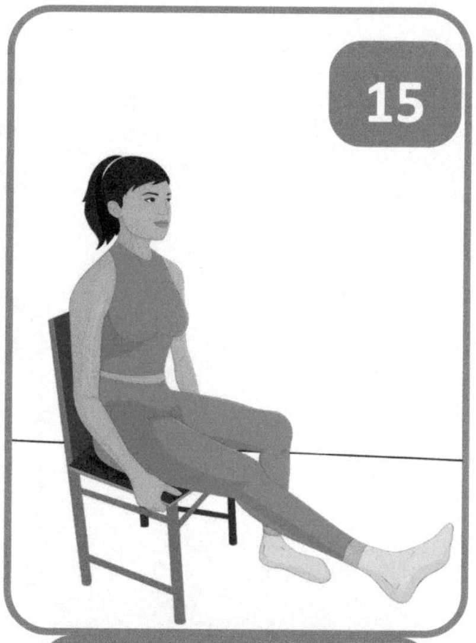

Chair Leg Extension

8 reps each side

Chair Glute Extension

8 reps each side

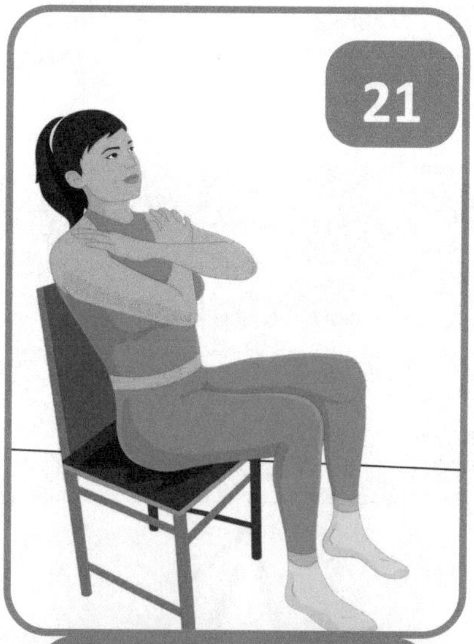

Chair Squat + Swing

10 reps

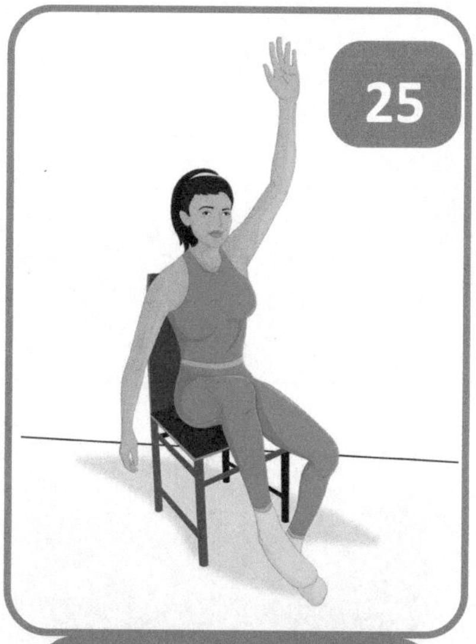

Chair Full March

30 seconds work

Day 2 - Perform it two times

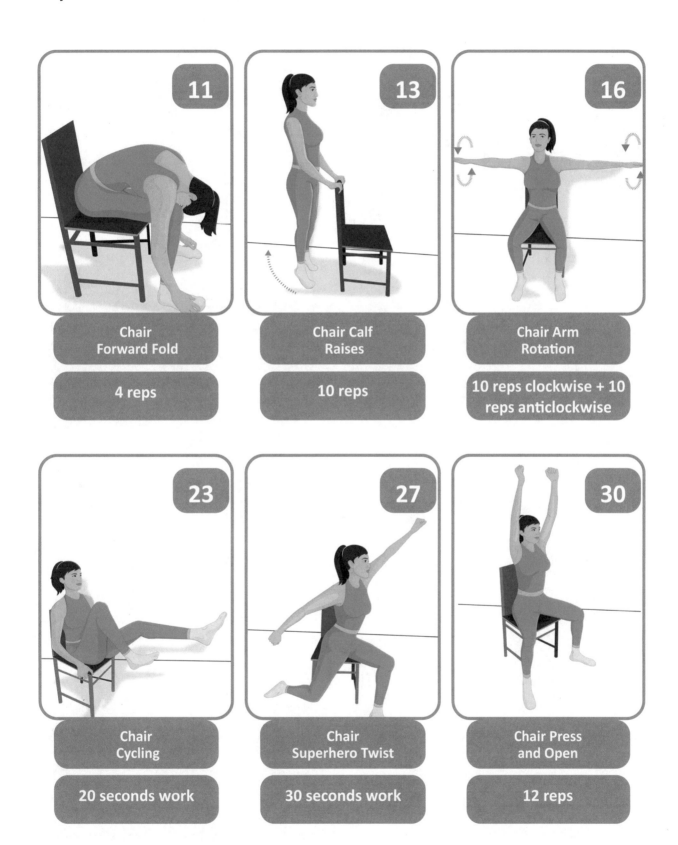

Chair
Forward Fold

4 reps

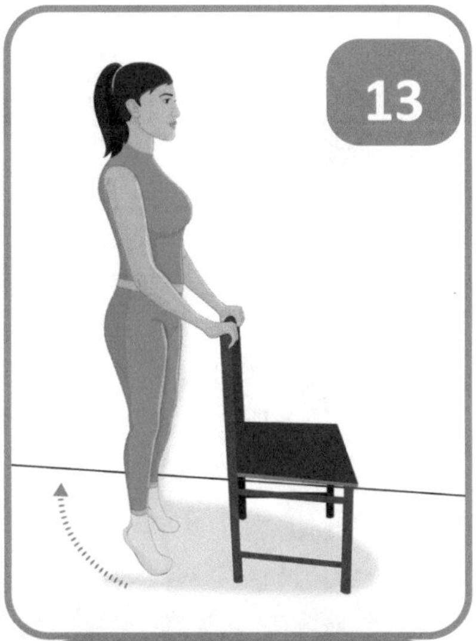

Chair Calf
Raises

10 reps

Chair Arm
Rotation

10 reps clockwise + 10 reps anticlockwise

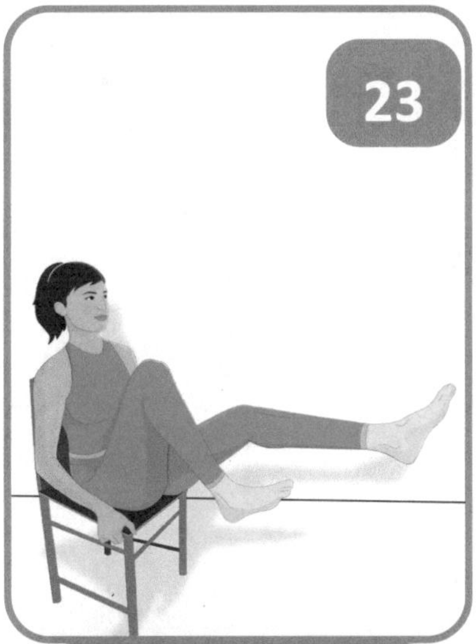

Chair
Cycling

20 seconds work

Chair
Superhero Twist

30 seconds work

Chair Press
and Open

12 reps

Day 3 - Perform it two times

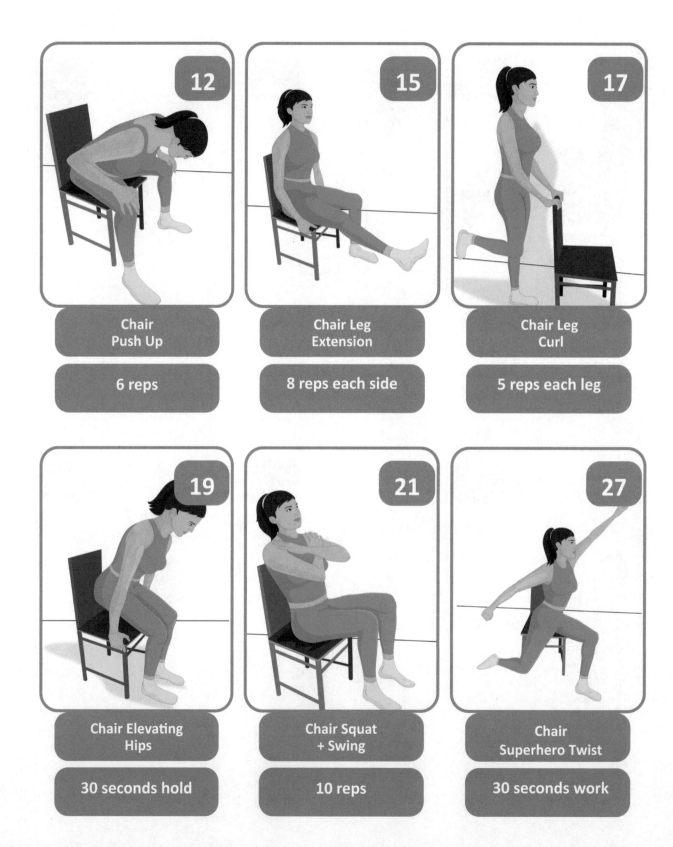

Chair
Push Up

6 reps

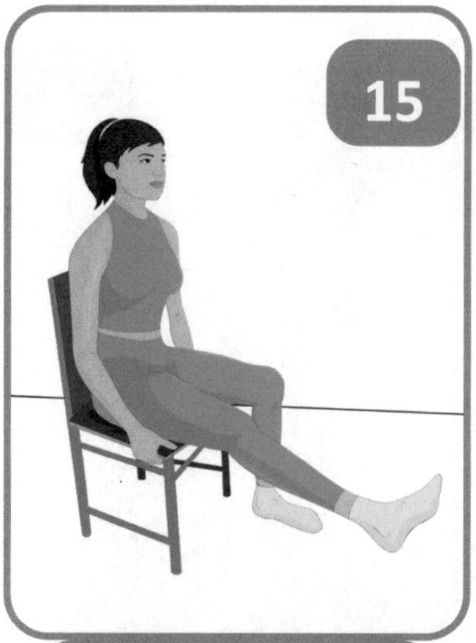

Chair Leg
Extension

8 reps each side

Chair Leg
Curl

5 reps each leg

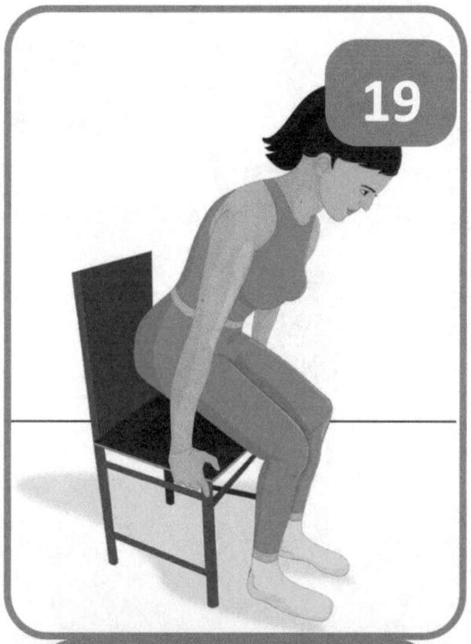

Chair Elevating
Hips

30 seconds hold

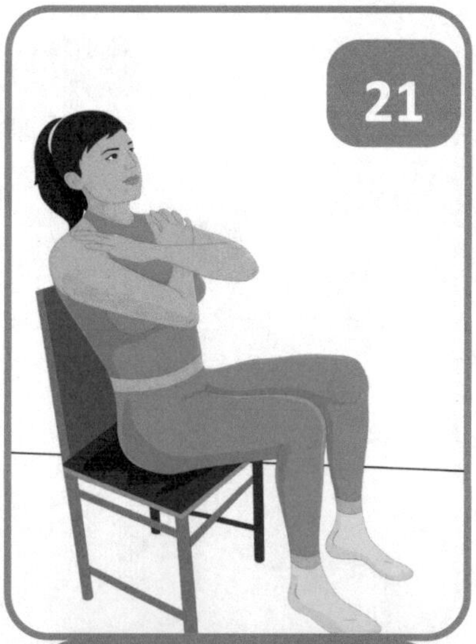

Chair Squat
+ Swing

10 reps

Chair
Superhero Twist

30 seconds work

Day 4 - Perform it two times

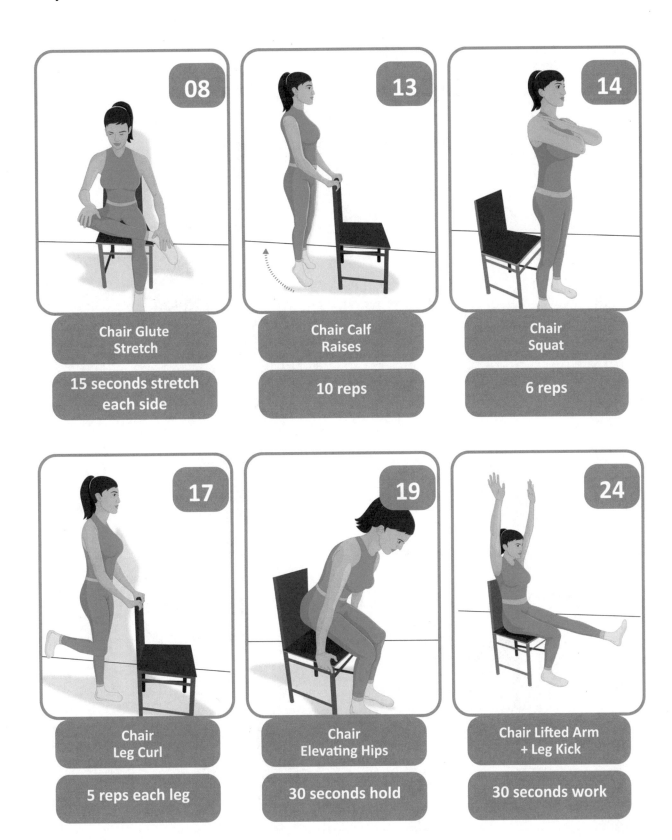

Chair Glute Stretch

15 seconds stretch each side

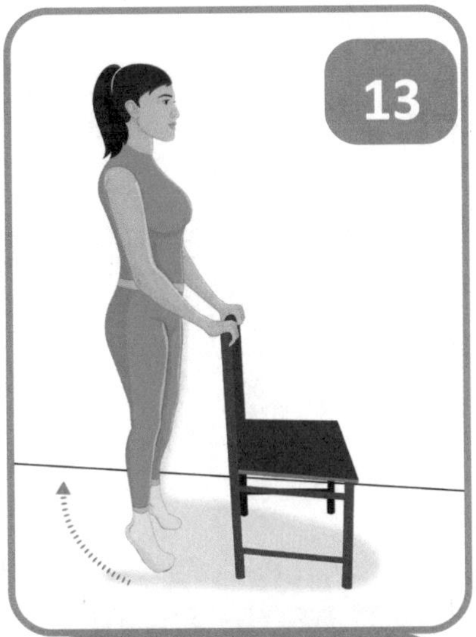

Chair Calf Raises

10 reps

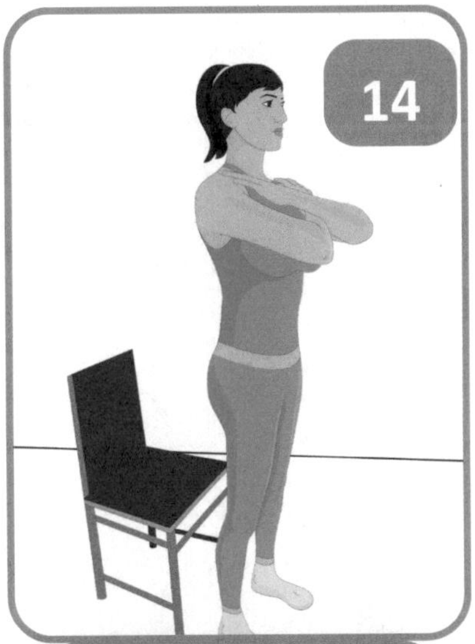

Chair Squat

6 reps

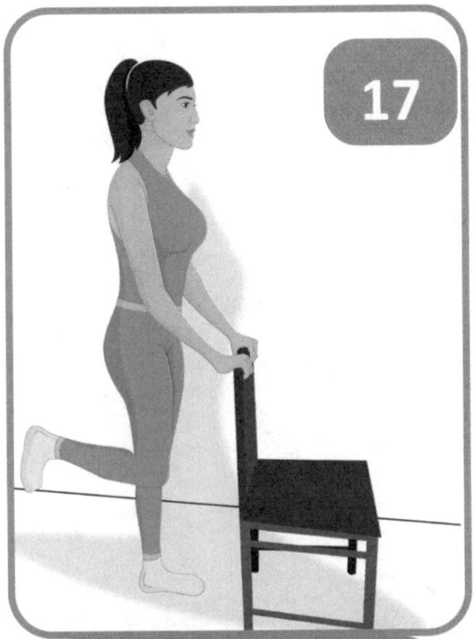

Chair Leg Curl

5 reps each leg

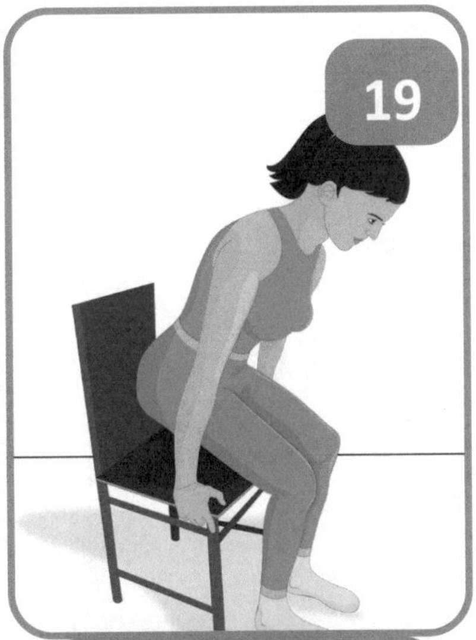

Chair Elevating Hips

30 seconds hold

Chair Lifted Arm + Leg Kick

30 seconds work

Day 5 - Perform it two times

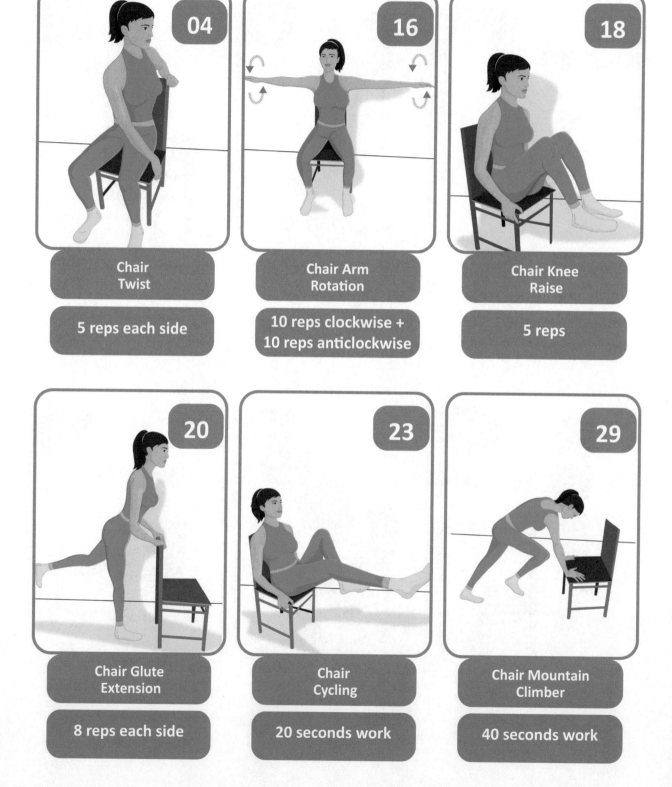

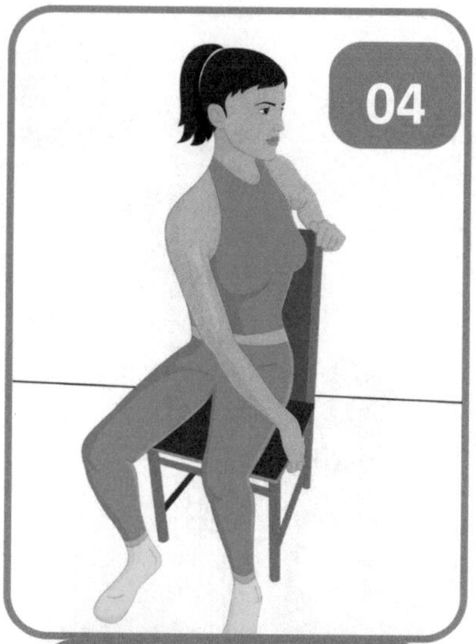

Chair Twist

5 reps each side

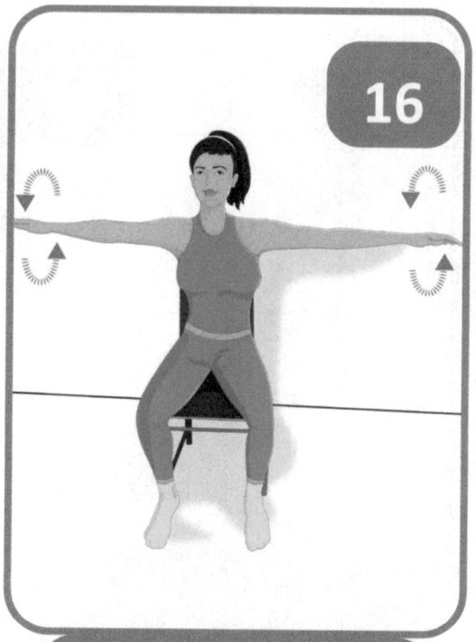

Chair Arm Rotation

10 reps clockwise +
10 reps anticlockwise

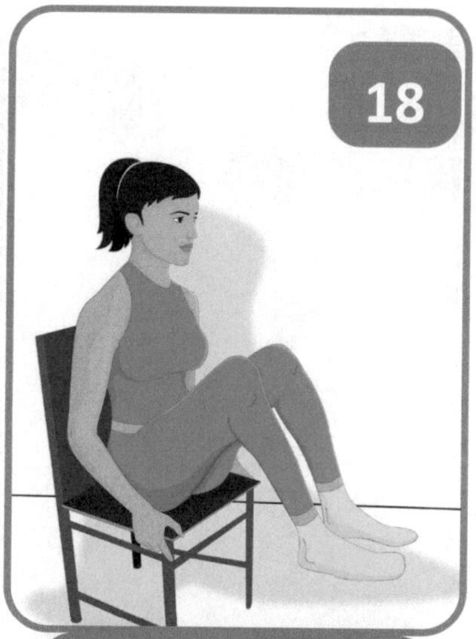

Chair Knee Raise

5 reps

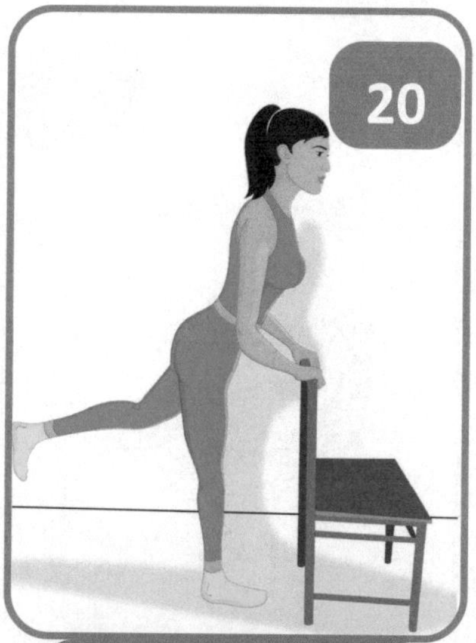

Chair Glute Extension

8 reps each side

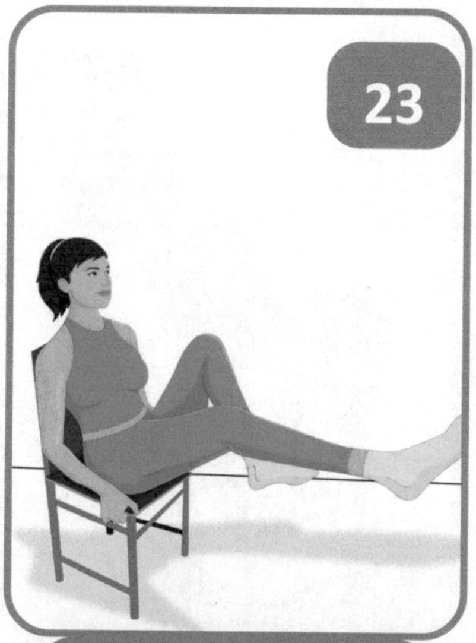

Chair Cycling

20 seconds work

Chair Mountain Climber

40 seconds work

Day 6 - Perform it two times

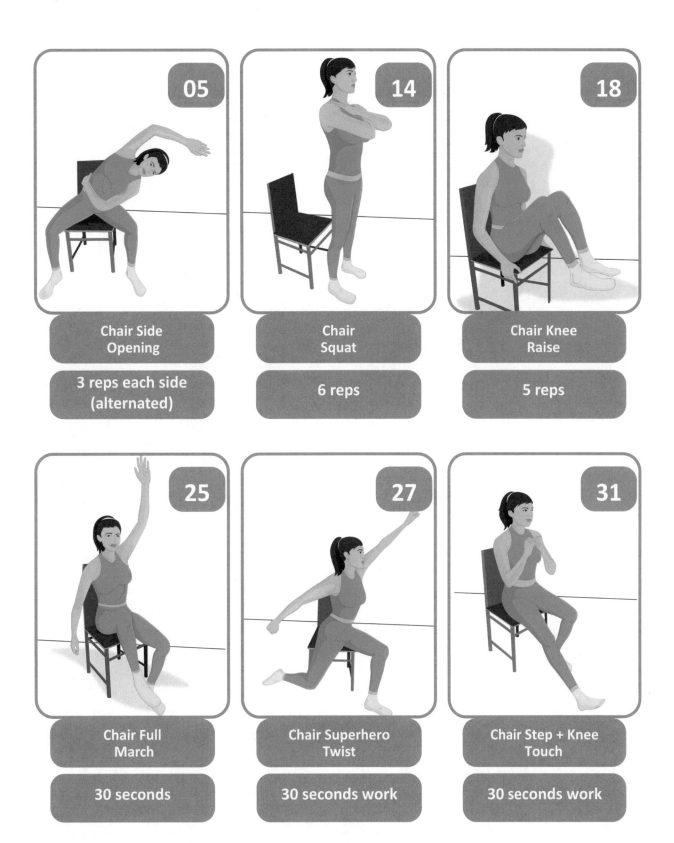

Chair Side Opening

3 reps each side (alternated)

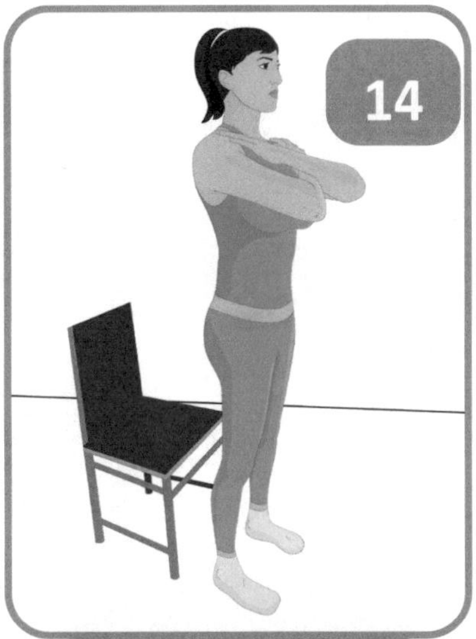

Chair Squat

6 reps

Chair Knee Raise

5 reps

Chair Full March

30 seconds

Chair Superhero Twist

30 seconds work

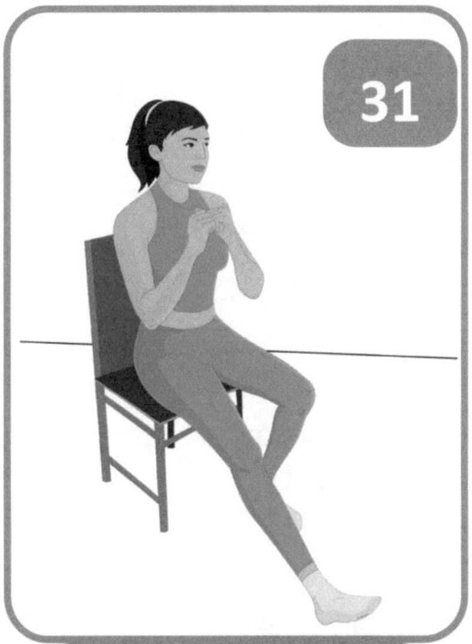

Chair Step + Knee Touch

30 seconds work

Day 7 - Perform it two times - Stretching Only

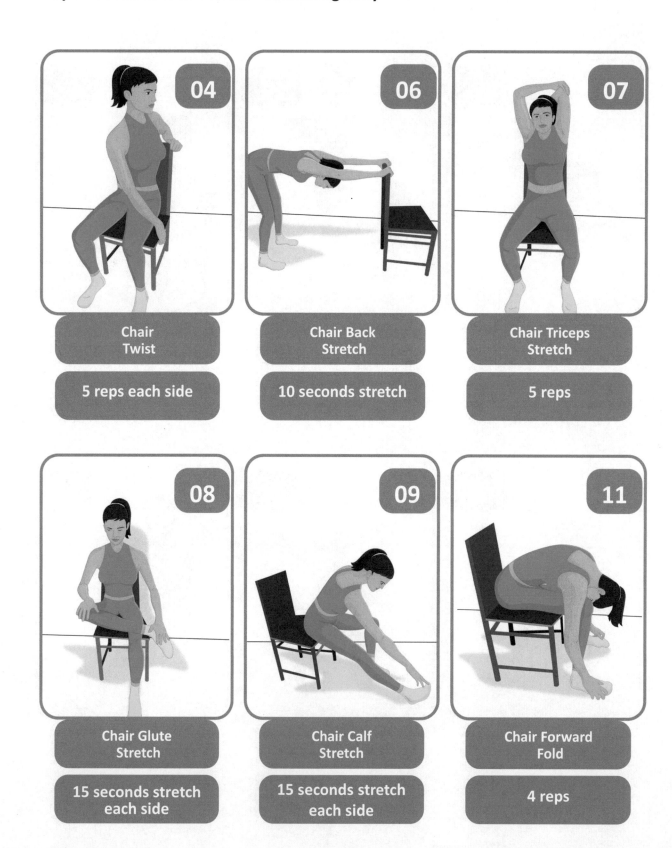

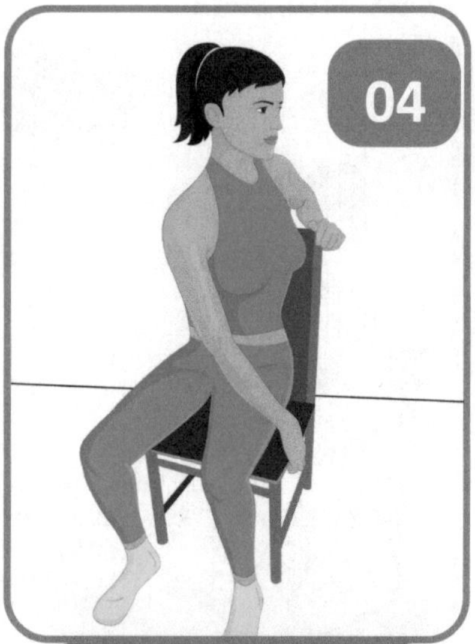

Chair Twist

5 reps each side

Chair Back Stretch

10 seconds stretch

Chair Triceps Stretch

5 reps

Chair Glute Stretch

15 seconds stretch each side

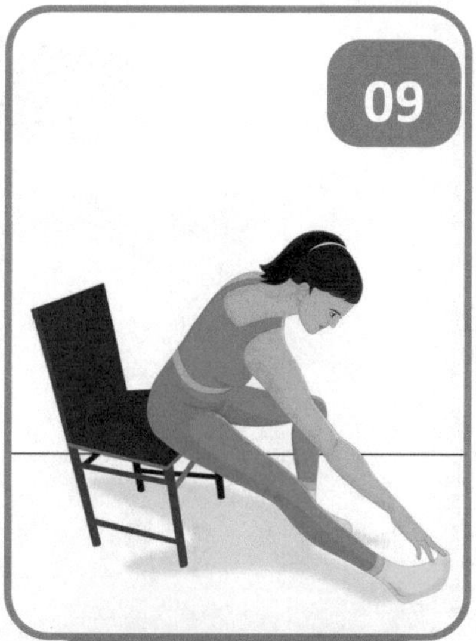

Chair Calf Stretch

15 seconds stretch each side

Chair Forward Fold

4 reps

Day 8 - Perform it three times

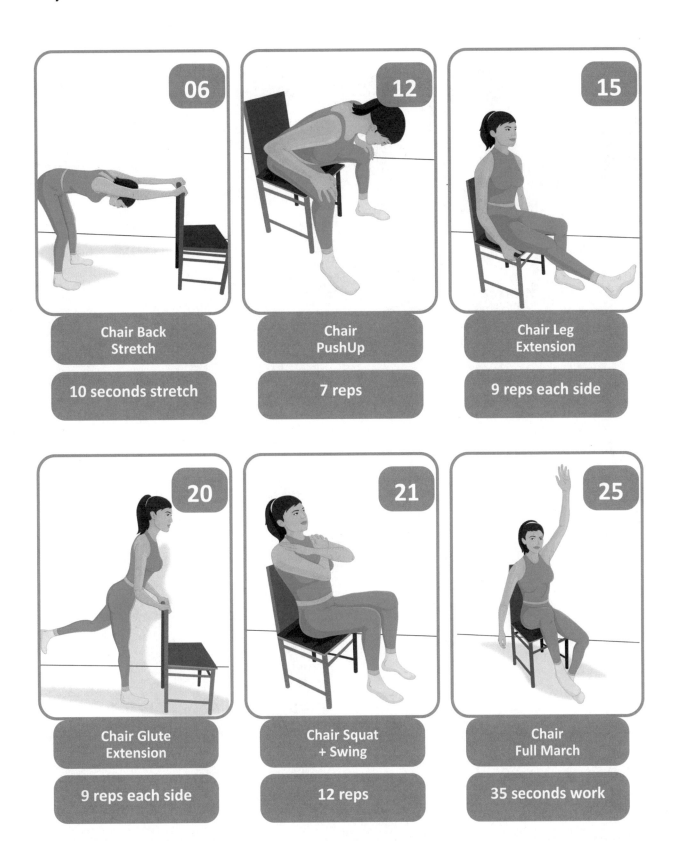

Chair Back Stretch

10 seconds stretch

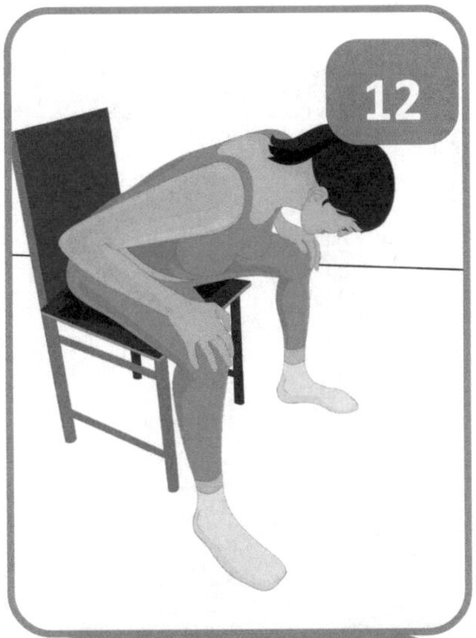

Chair PushUp

7 reps

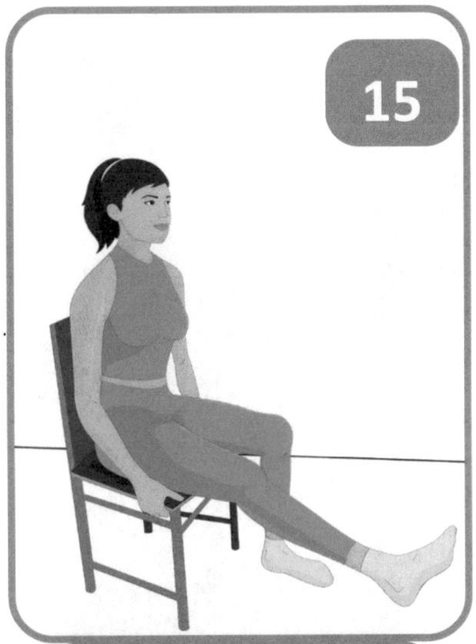

Chair Leg Extension

9 reps each side

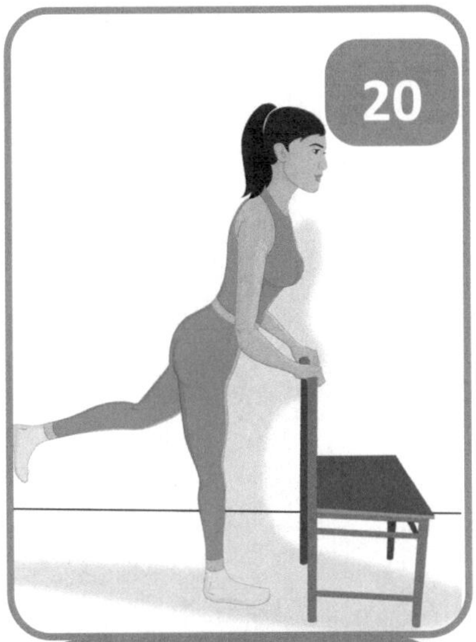

Chair Glute Extension

9 reps each side

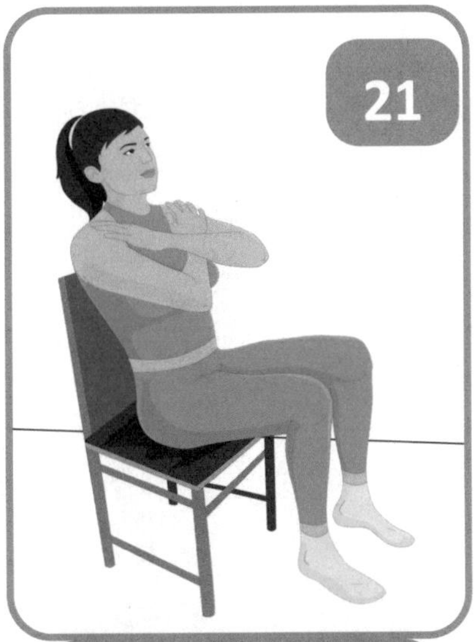

Chair Squat + Swing

12 reps

Chair Full March

35 seconds work

Day 9 - Perform it three times

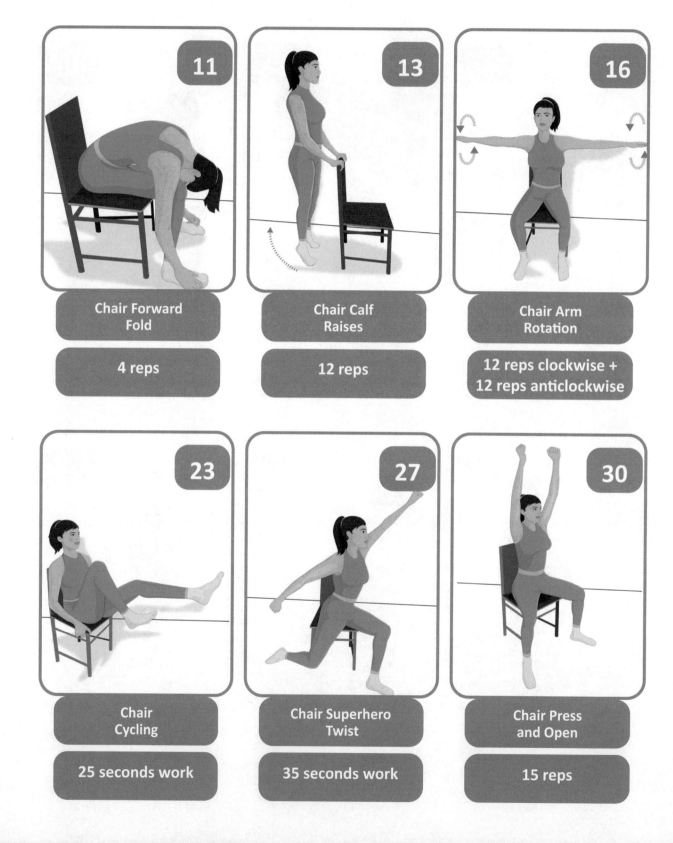

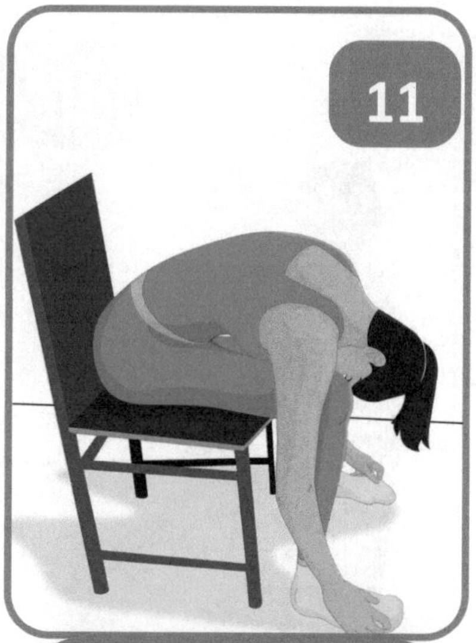

Chair Forward Fold

4 reps

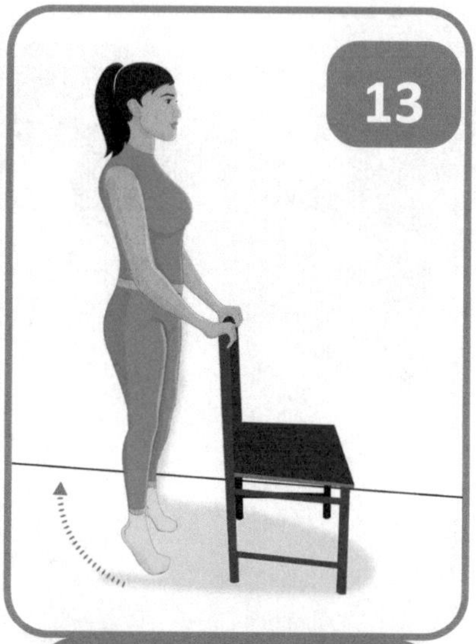

Chair Calf Raises

12 reps

Chair Arm Rotation

12 reps clockwise +
12 reps anticlockwise

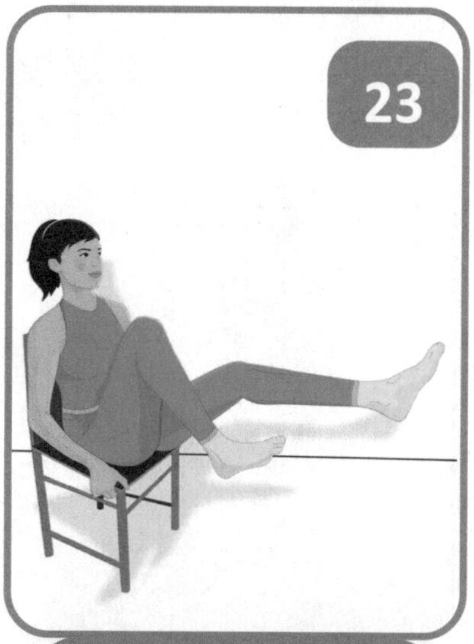

Chair Cycling

25 seconds work

Chair Superhero Twist

35 seconds work

Chair Press and Open

15 reps

Day 10 - Perform it three times

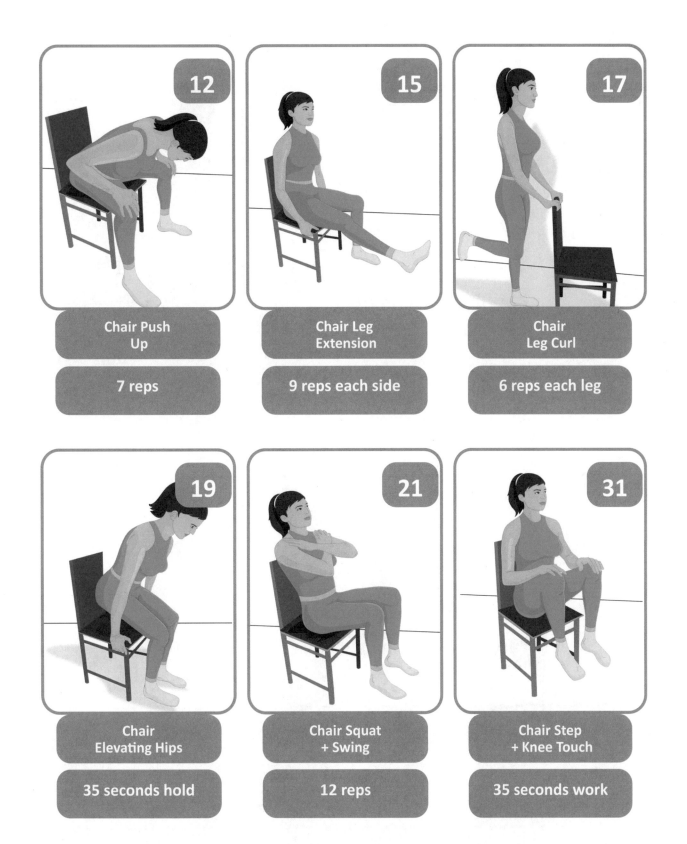

Chair Push Up

7 reps

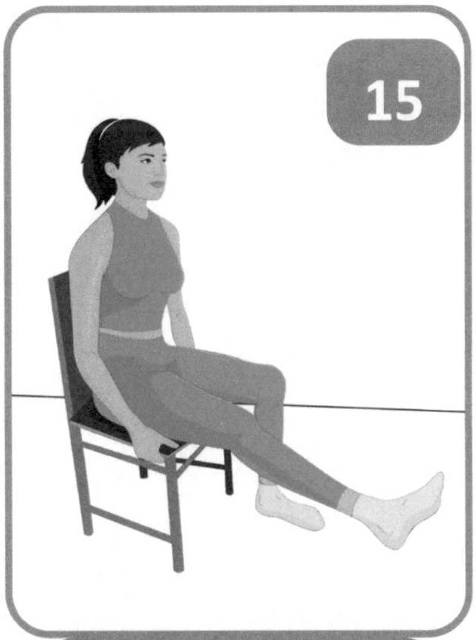

Chair Leg Extension

9 reps each side

Chair Leg Curl

6 reps each leg

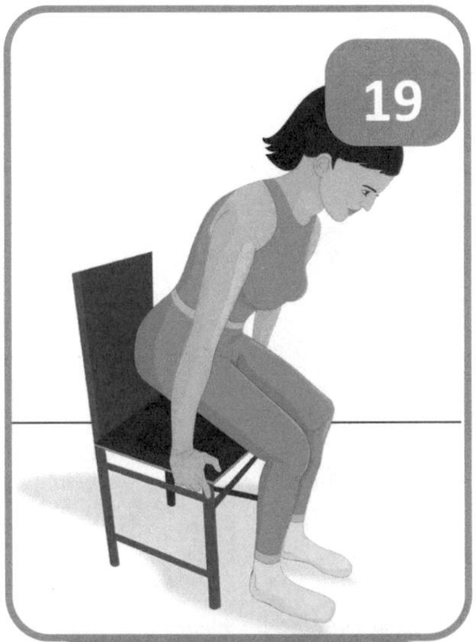

Chair Elevating Hips

35 seconds hold

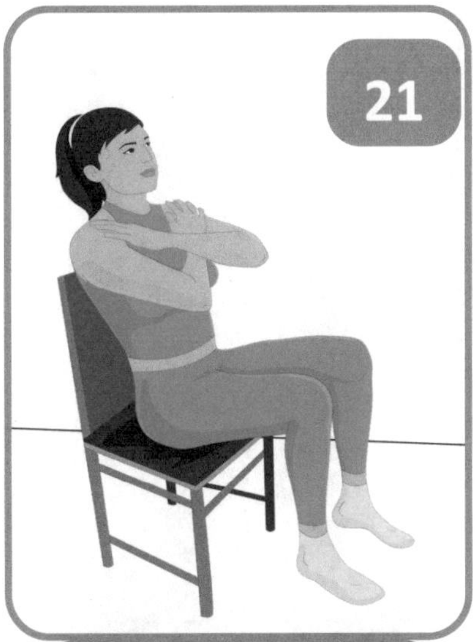

Chair Squat + Swing

12 reps

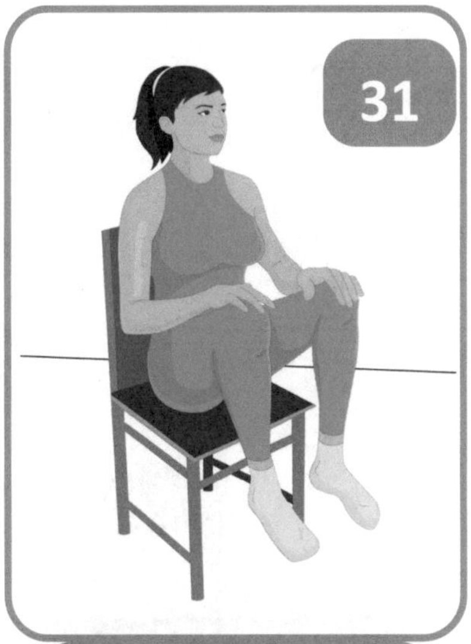

Chair Step + Knee Touch

35 seconds work

Day 11 - Perform it three times

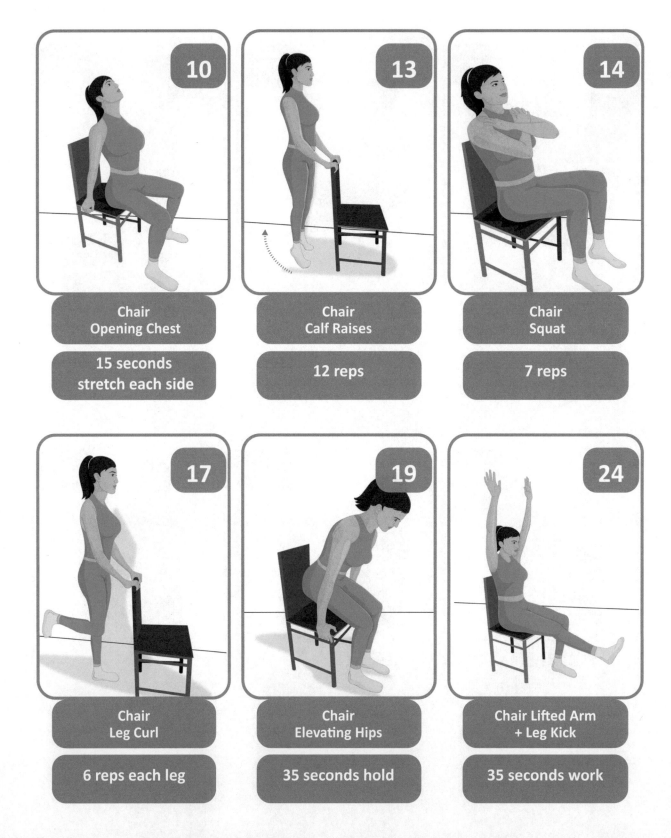

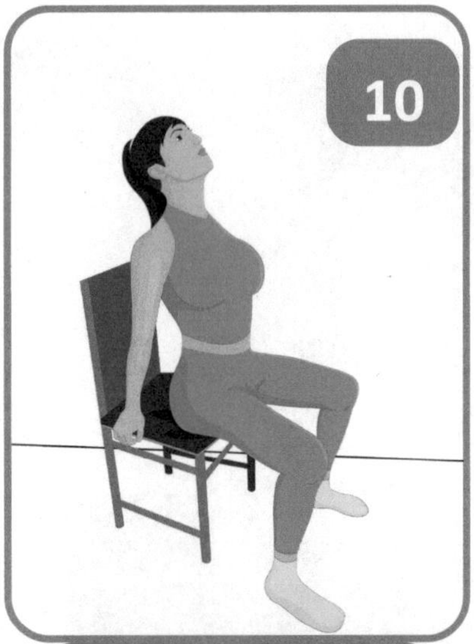

Chair
Opening Chest

15 seconds
stretch each side

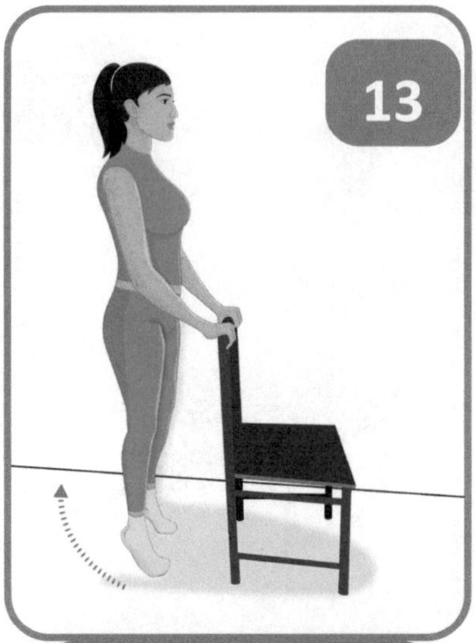

Chair
Calf Raises

12 reps

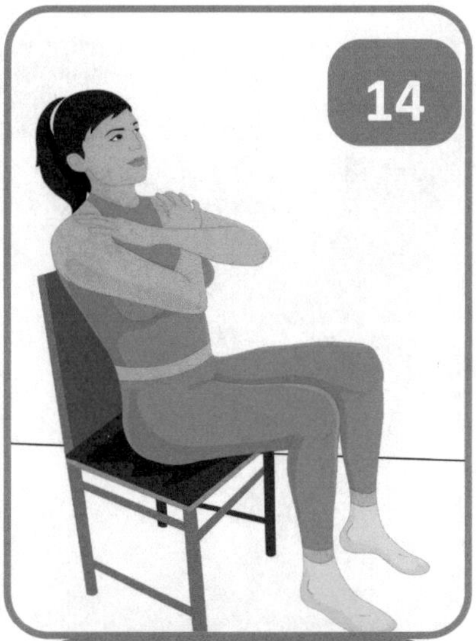

Chair
Squat

7 reps

Chair
Leg Curl

6 reps each leg

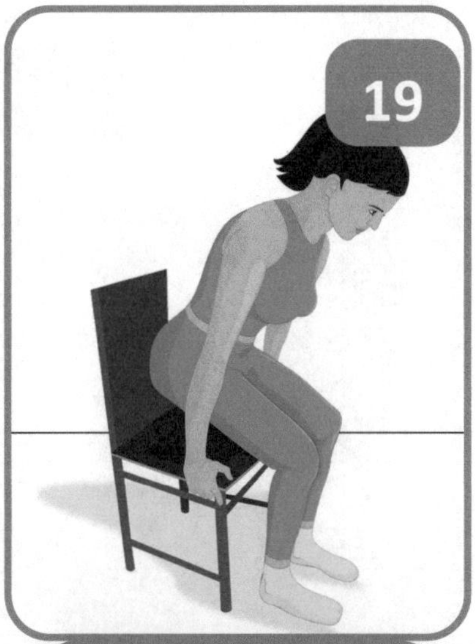

Chair
Elevating Hips

35 seconds hold

Chair Lifted Arm
+ Leg Kick

35 seconds work

Day 12 - Perform it three times

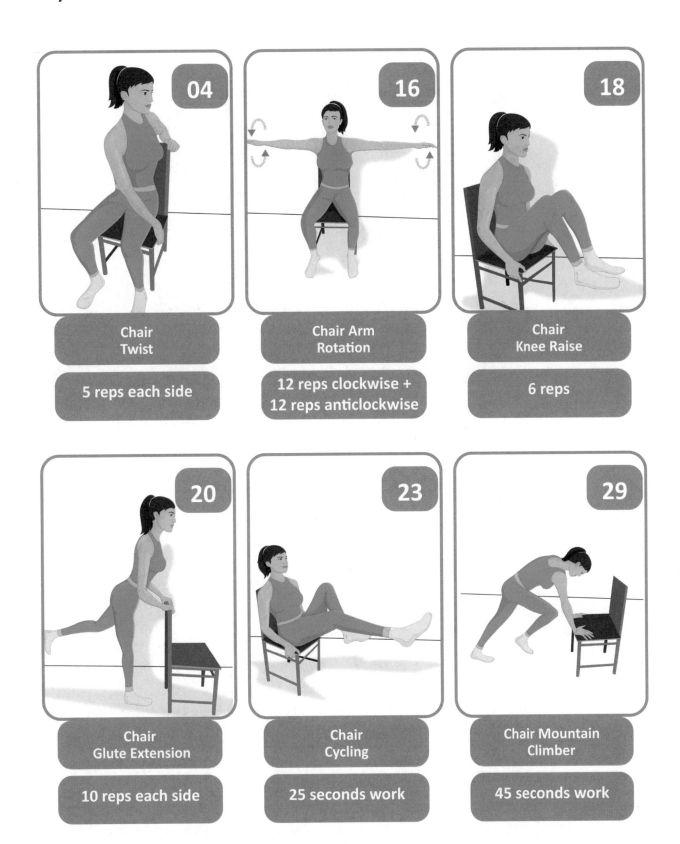

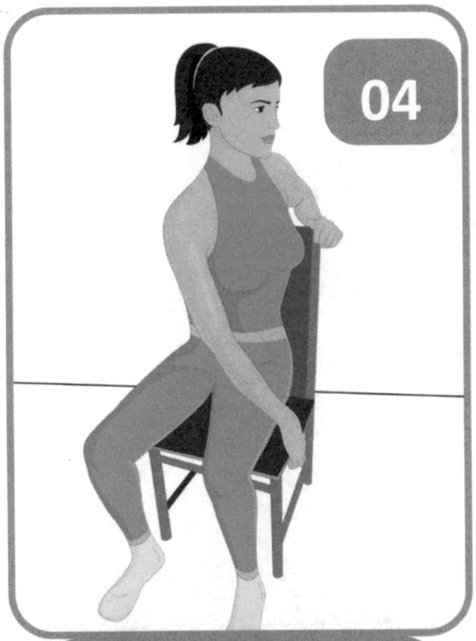

Chair Twist

5 reps each side

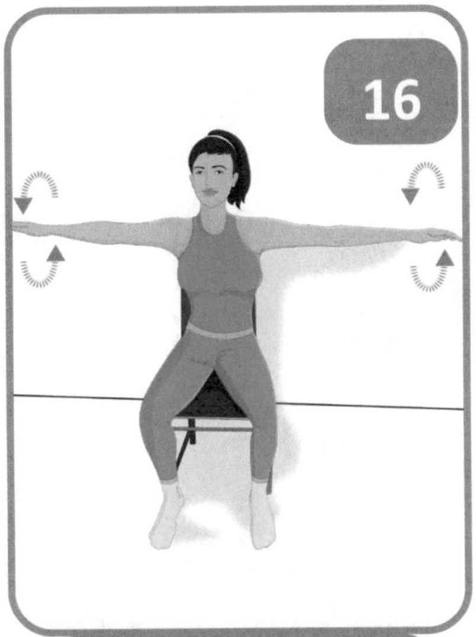

Chair Arm Rotation

12 reps clockwise +
12 reps anticlockwise

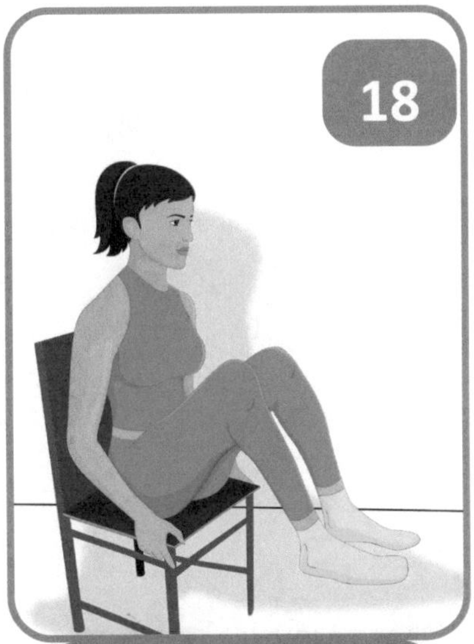

Chair Knee Raise

6 reps

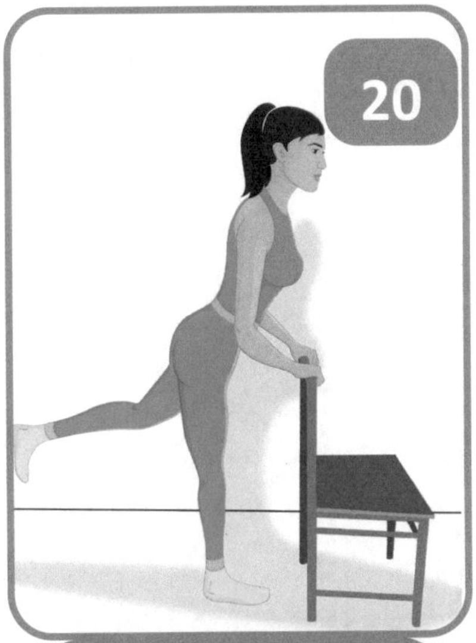

Chair Glute Extension

10 reps each side

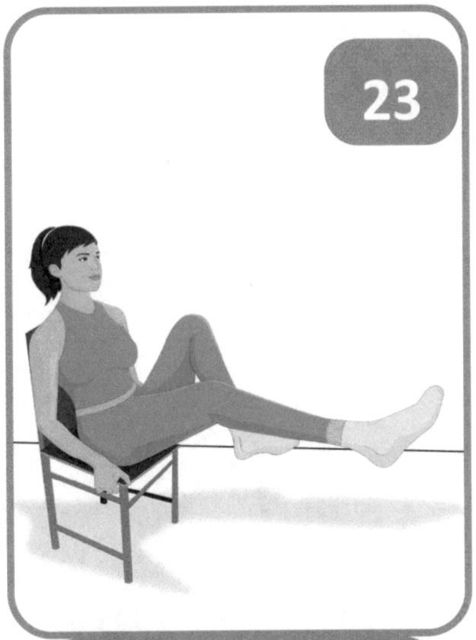

Chair Cycling

25 seconds work

Chair Mountain Climber

45 seconds work

Day 13 - Perform it three times

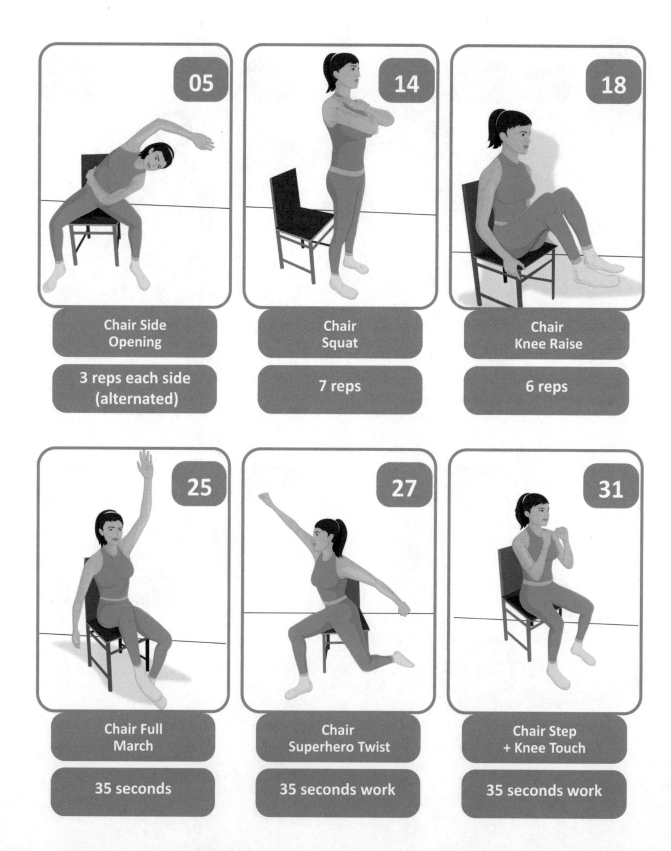

Chair Side Opening

3 reps each side (alternated)

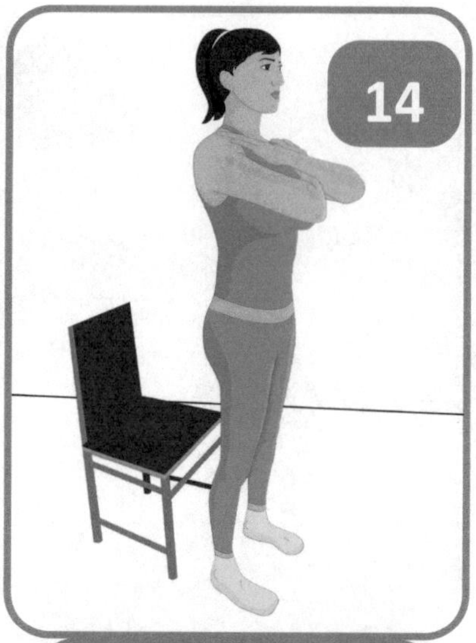

Chair Squat

7 reps

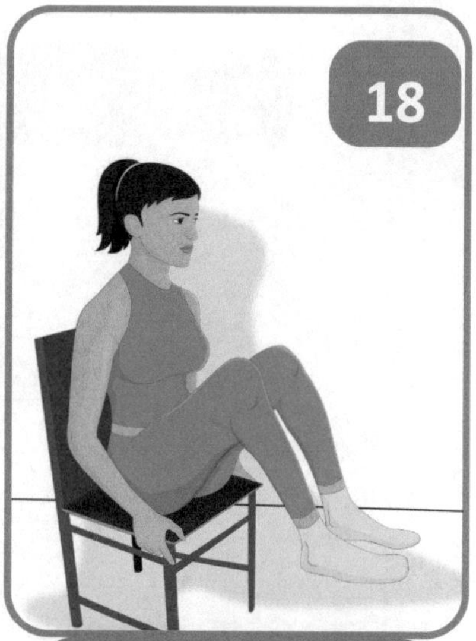

Chair Knee Raise

6 reps

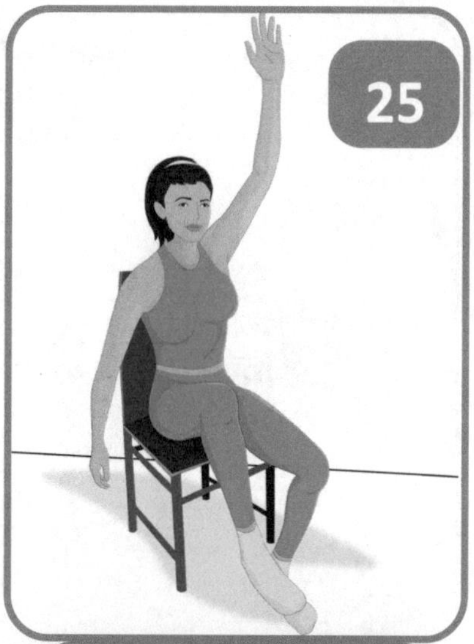

Chair Full March

35 seconds

Chair Superhero Twist

35 seconds work

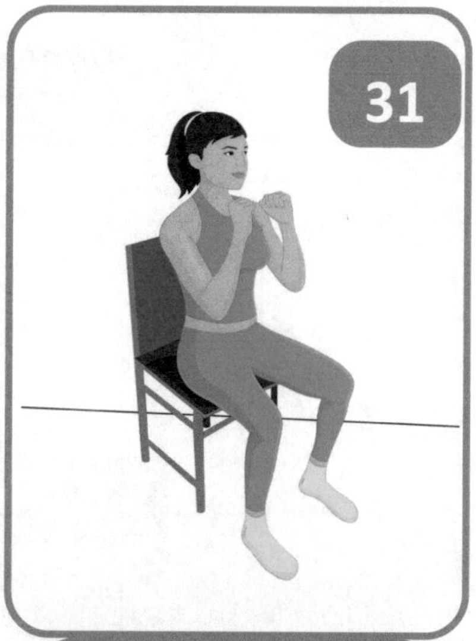

Chair Step + Knee Touch

35 seconds work

Day 14 - Perform it two times - Stretching Only

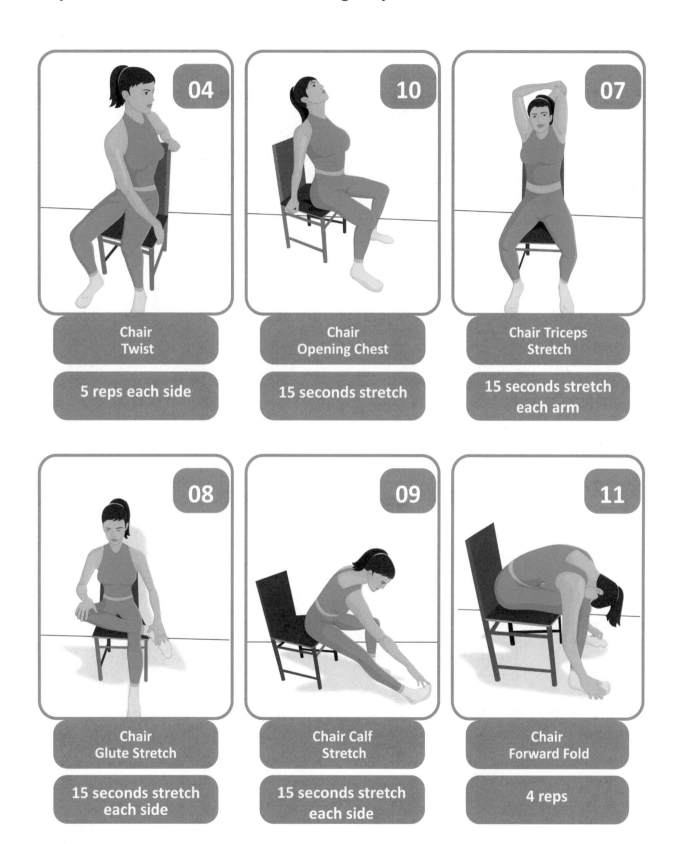

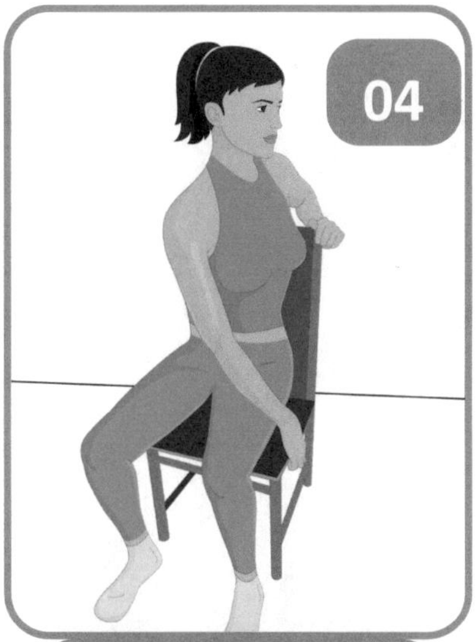

Chair Twist

5 reps each side

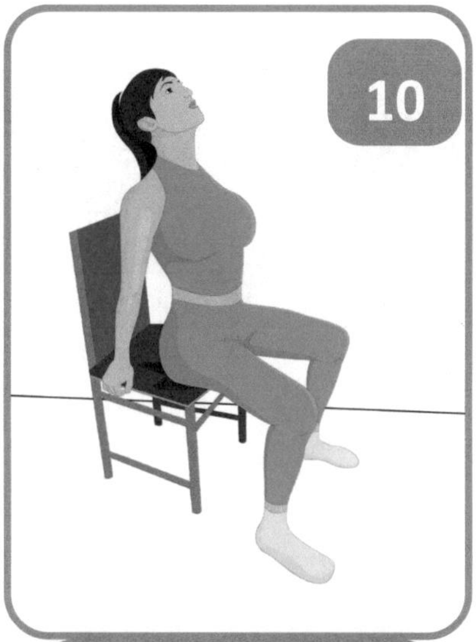

Chair Opening Chest

15 seconds stretch

Chair Triceps Stretch

15 seconds stretch each arm

Chair Glute Stretch

15 seconds stretch each side

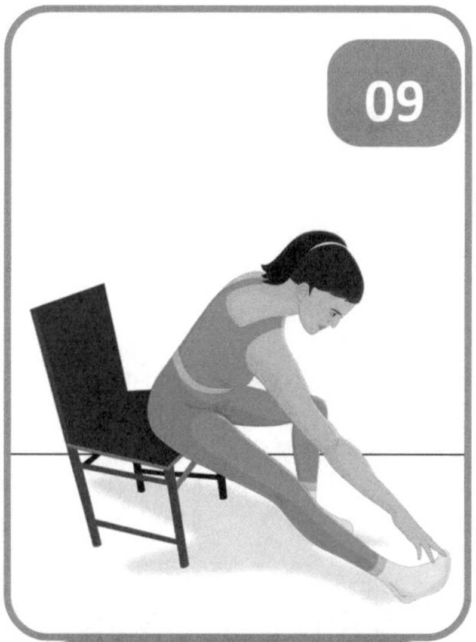

Chair Calf Stretch

15 seconds stretch each side

Chair Forward Fold

4 reps

Day 15 - Perform it three times

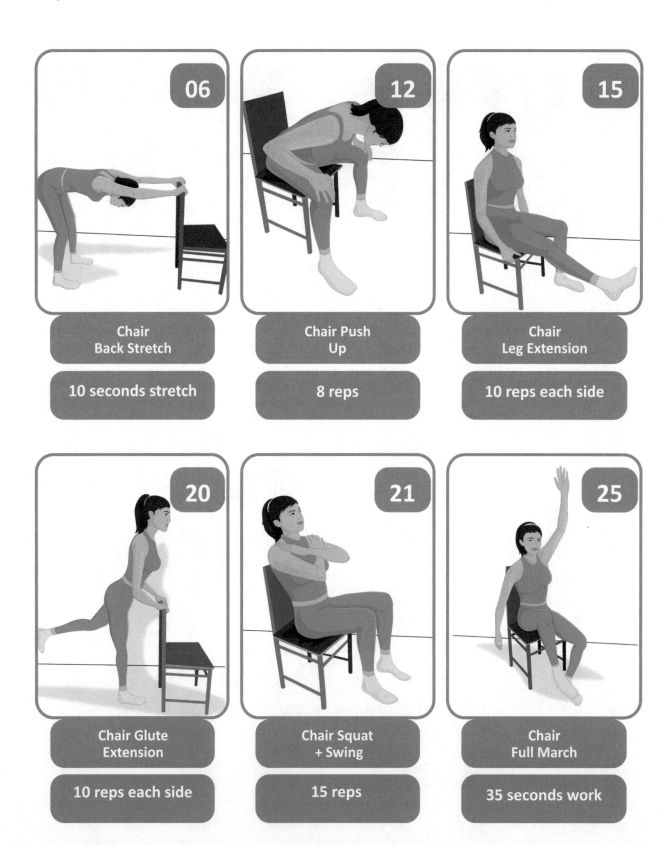

Chair
Back Stretch

10 seconds stretch

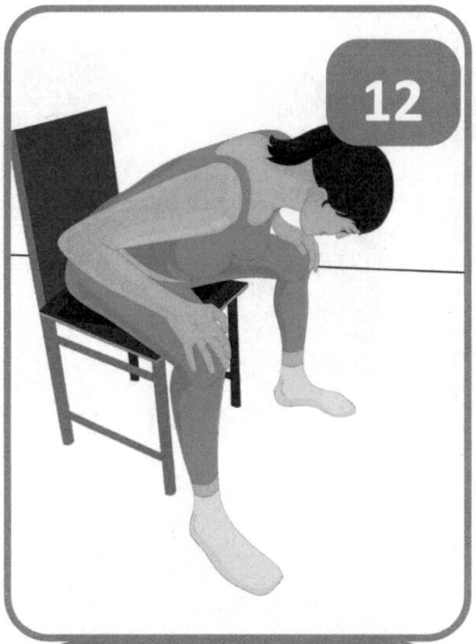

Chair Push
Up

8 reps

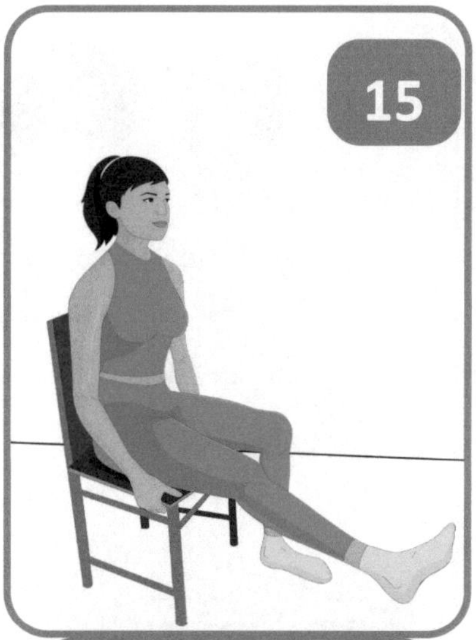

Chair
Leg Extension

10 reps each side

Chair Glute
Extension

10 reps each side

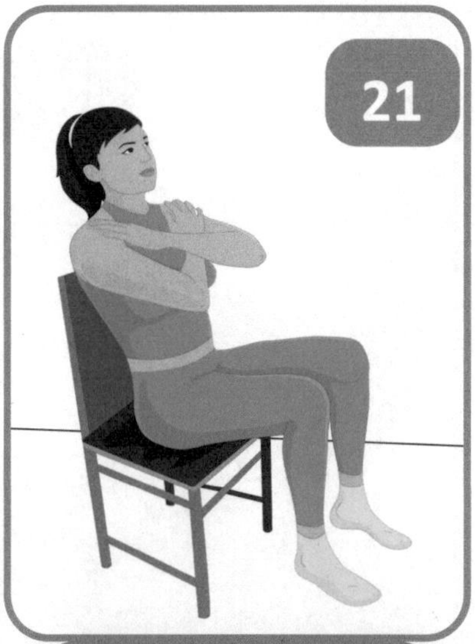

Chair Squat
+ Swing

15 reps

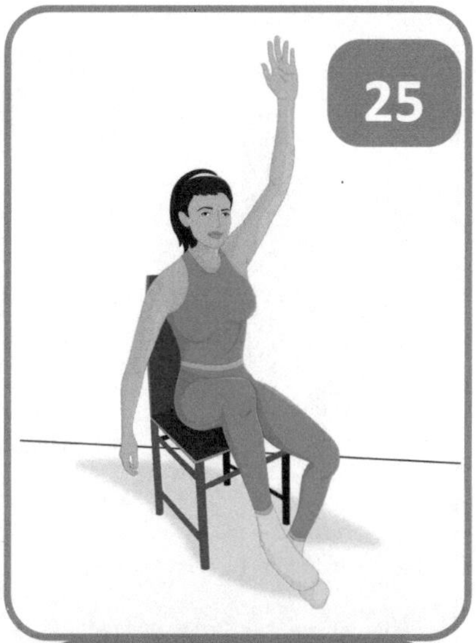

Chair
Full March

35 seconds work

Day 16 - Perform it three times

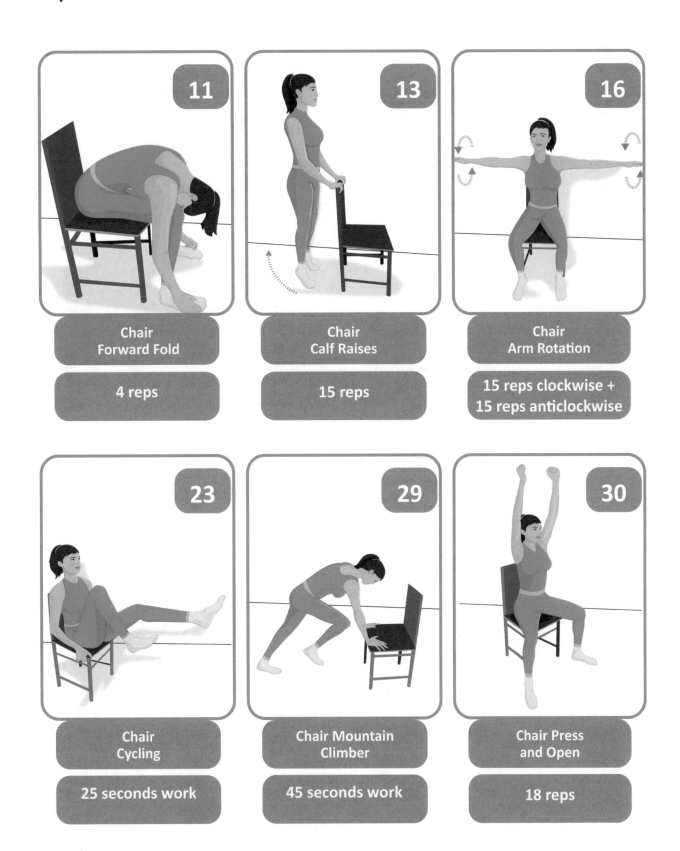

Chair
Forward Fold

4 reps

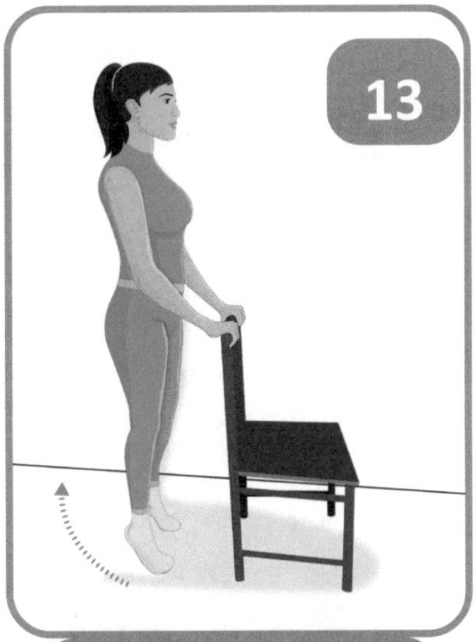

Chair
Calf Raises

15 reps

Chair
Arm Rotation

15 reps clockwise +
15 reps anticlockwise

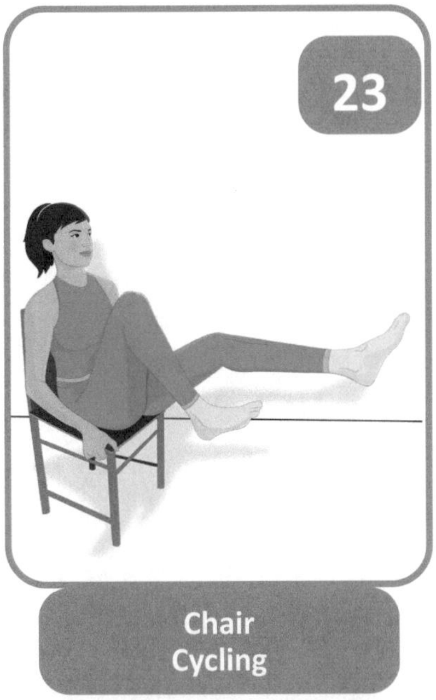

Chair
Cycling

25 seconds work

Chair Mountain
Climber

45 seconds work

Chair Press
and Open

18 reps

Day 17 - Perform it three times

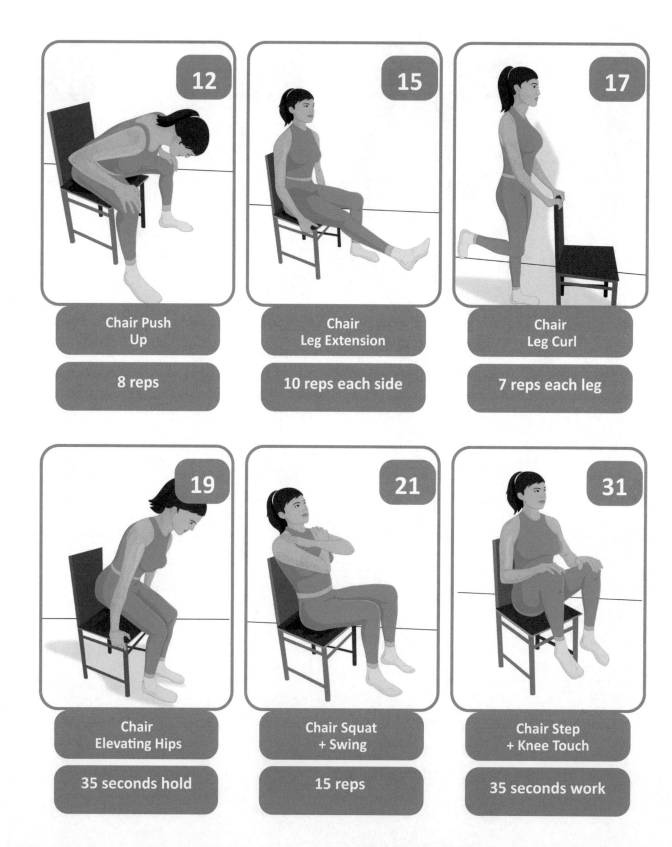

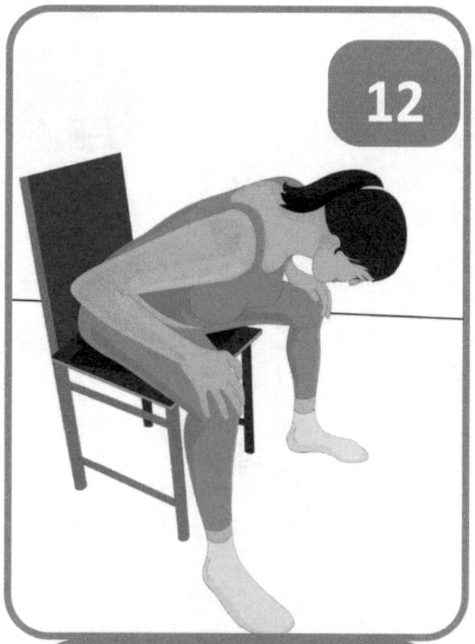

Chair Push Up

8 reps

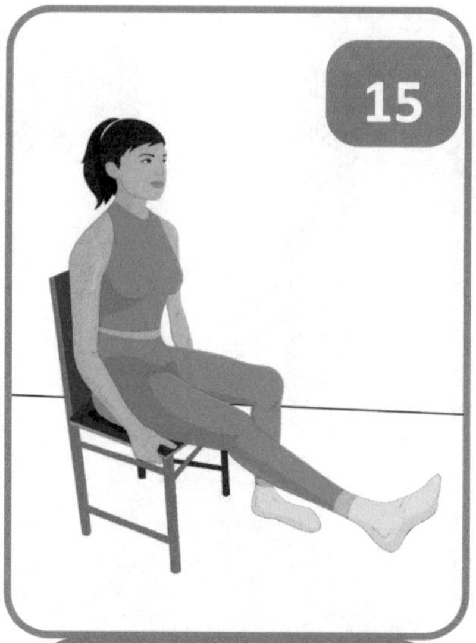

Chair Leg Extension

10 reps each side

Chair Leg Curl

7 reps each leg

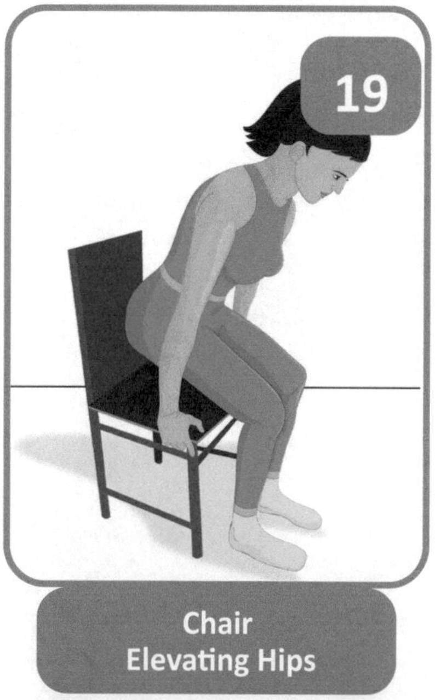

Chair Elevating Hips

35 seconds hold

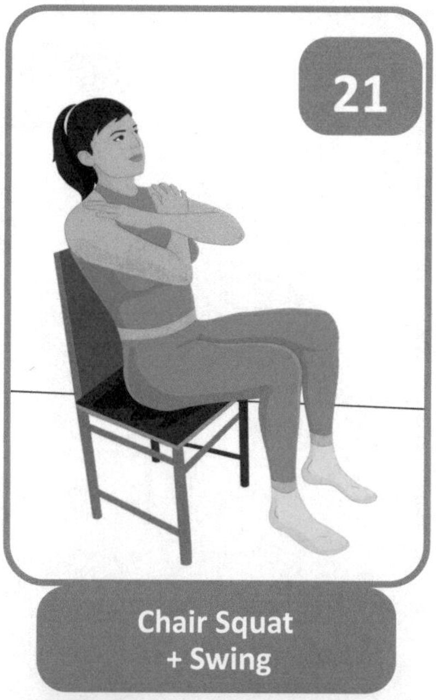

Chair Squat + Swing

15 reps

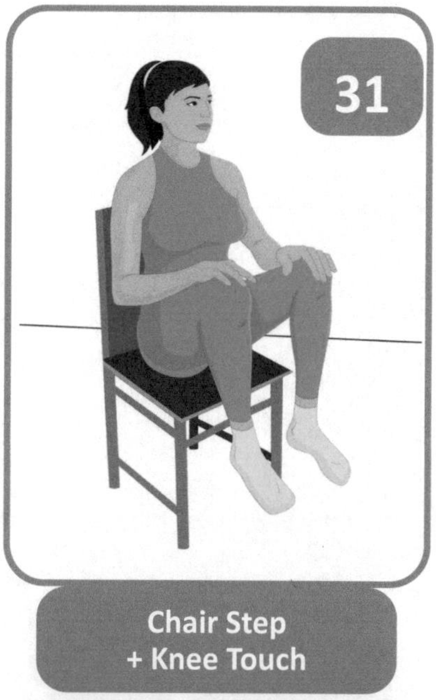

Chair Step + Knee Touch

35 seconds work

Day 18 - Perform it three times

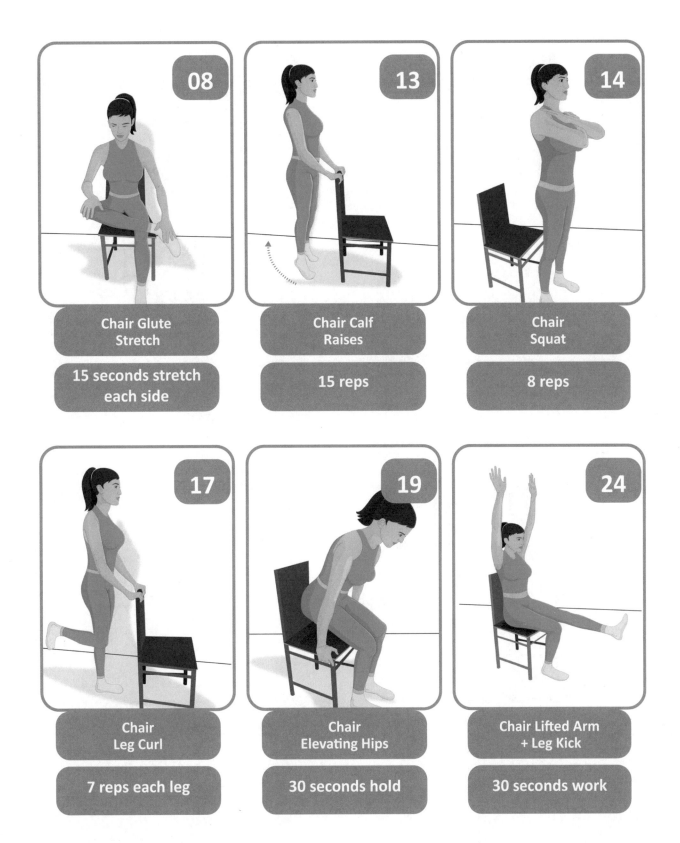

Chair Glute Stretch

15 seconds stretch each side

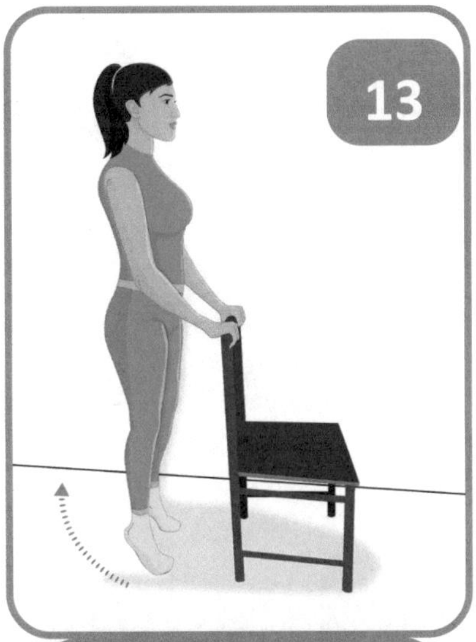

Chair Calf Raises

15 reps

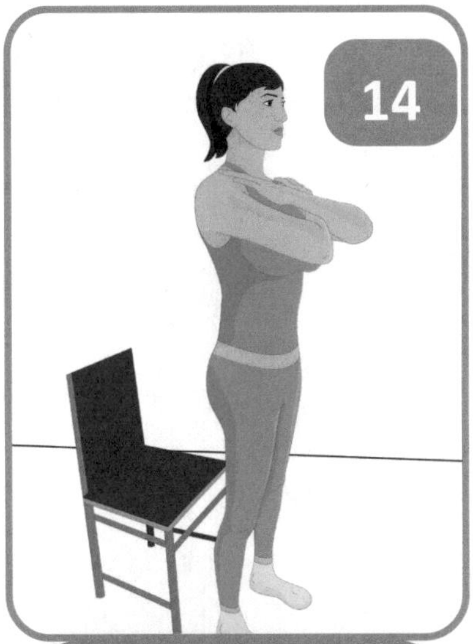

Chair Squat

8 reps

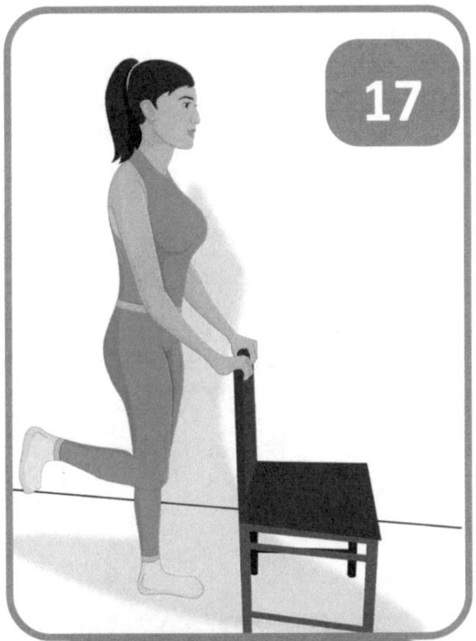

Chair Leg Curl

7 reps each leg

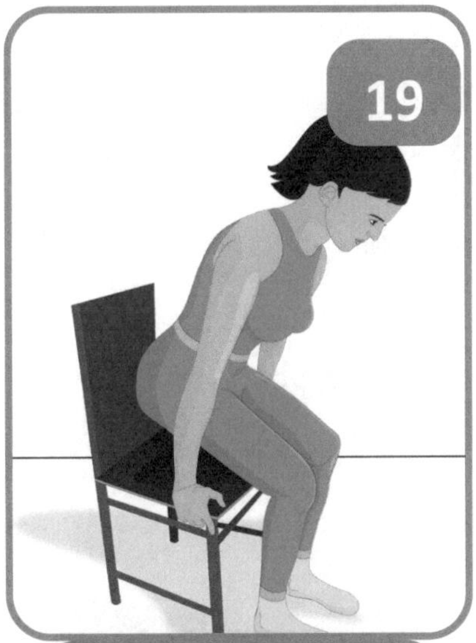

Chair Elevating Hips

30 seconds hold

Chair Lifted Arm + Leg Kick

30 seconds work

Day 19 - Perform it four times

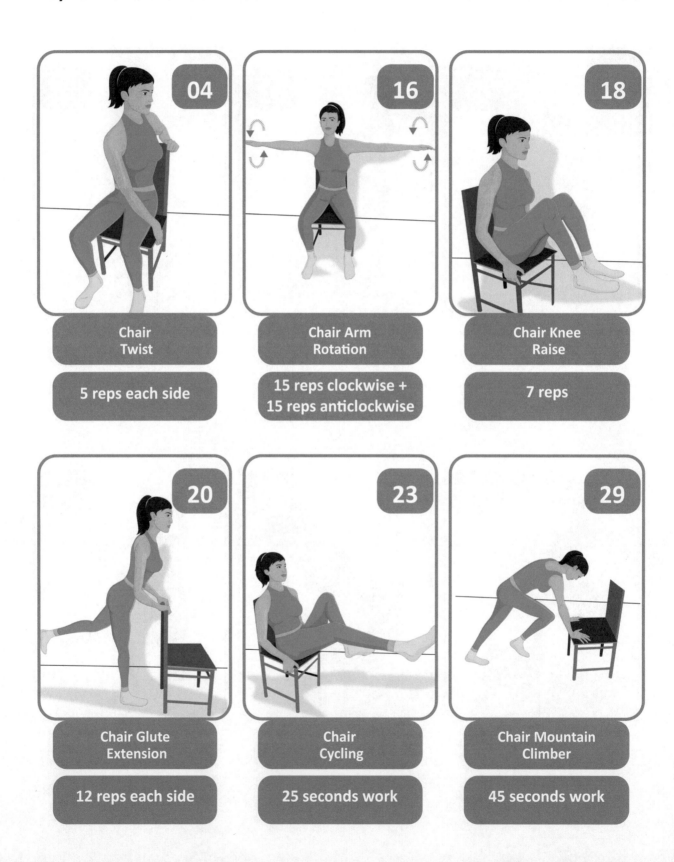

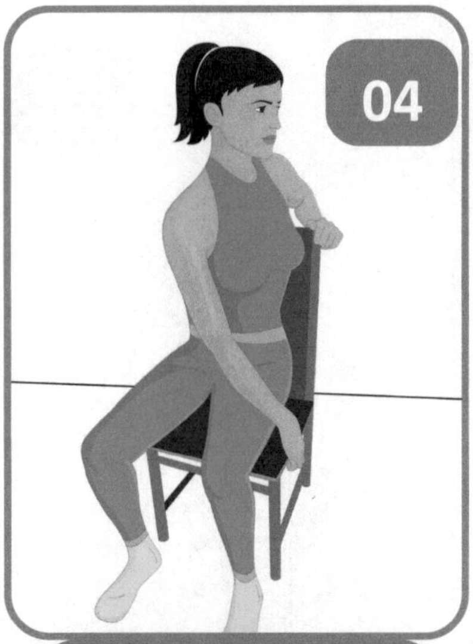

Chair Twist

5 reps each side

Chair Arm Rotation

15 reps clockwise + 15 reps anticlockwise

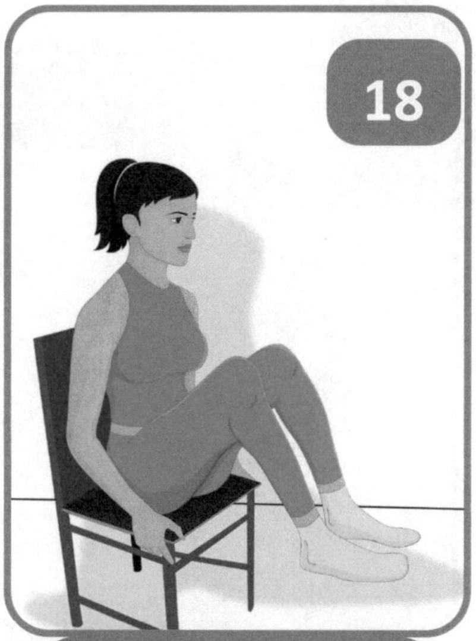

Chair Knee Raise

7 reps

Chair Glute Extension

12 reps each side

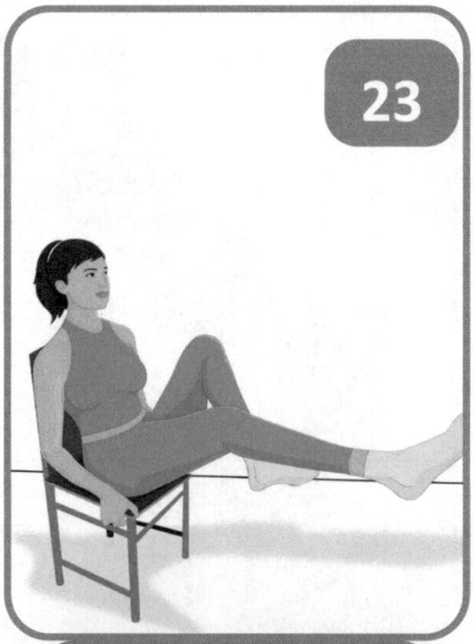

Chair Cycling

25 seconds work

Chair Mountain Climber

45 seconds work

Day 20 - Perform it four times

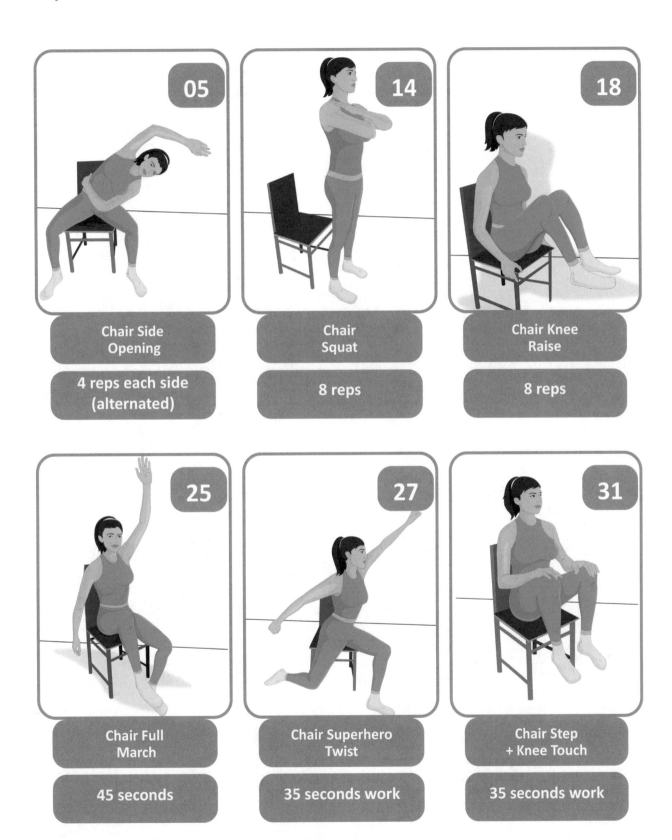

Chair Side Opening

4 reps each side (alternated)

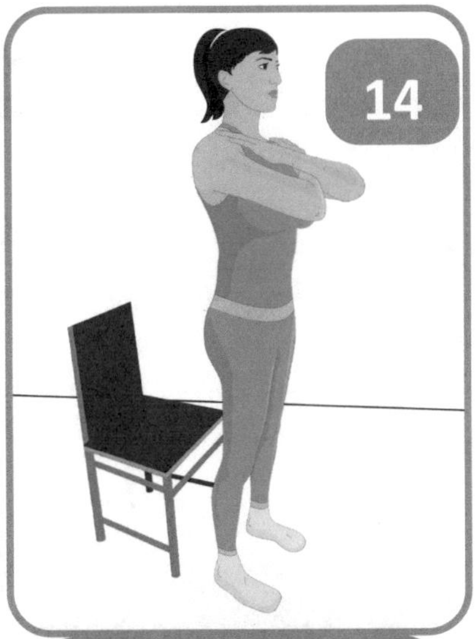

Chair Squat

8 reps

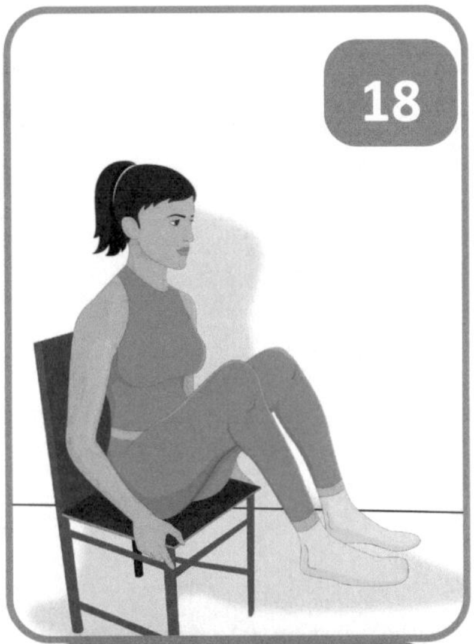

Chair Knee Raise

8 reps

Chair Full March

45 seconds

Chair Superhero Twist

35 seconds work

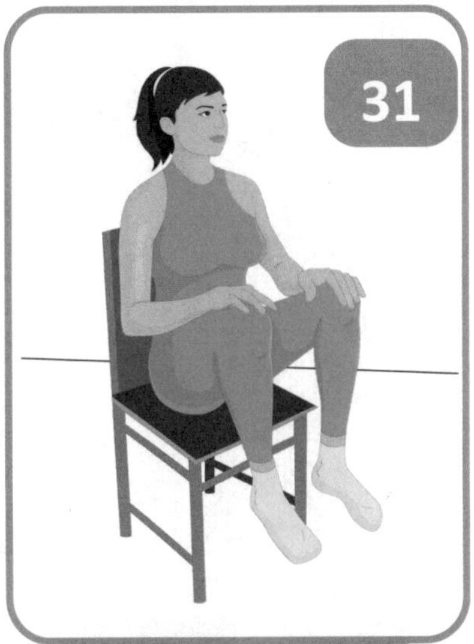

Chair Step + Knee Touch

35 seconds work

Day 21 - Perform it two times - Stretching only

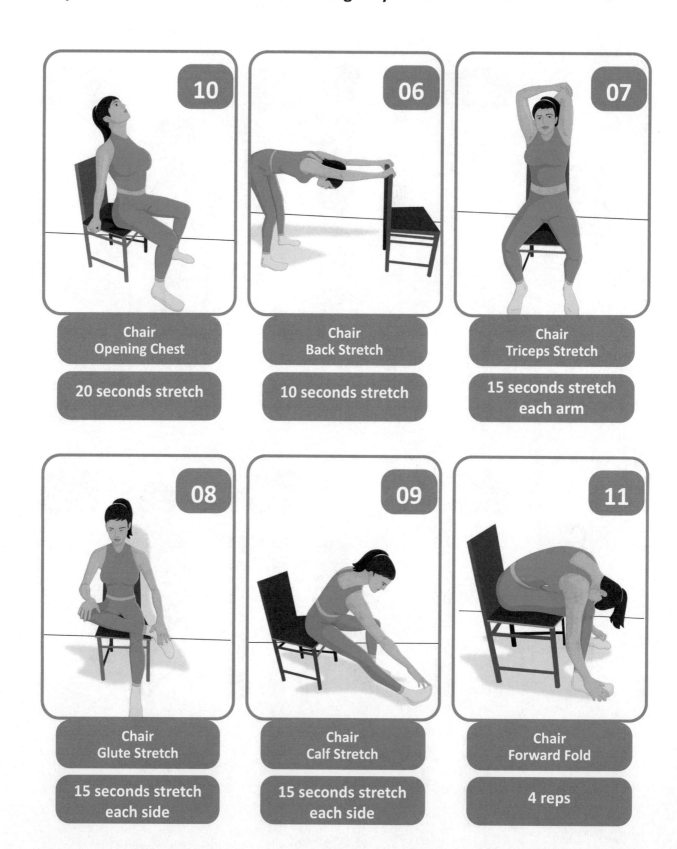

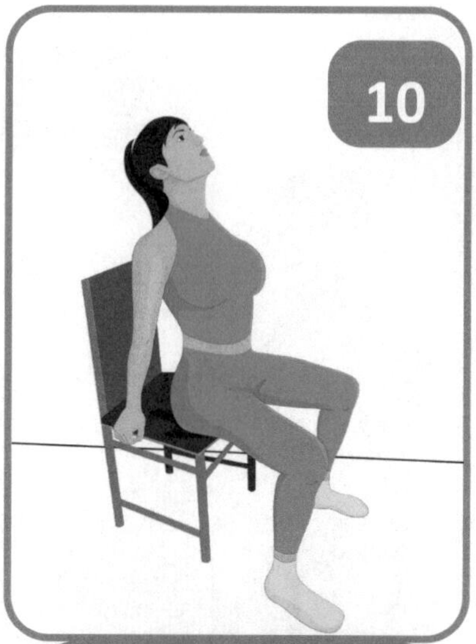

Chair
Opening Chest

20 seconds stretch

Chair
Back Stretch

10 seconds stretch

Chair
Triceps Stretch

15 seconds stretch each arm

Chair
Glute Stretch

15 seconds stretch each side

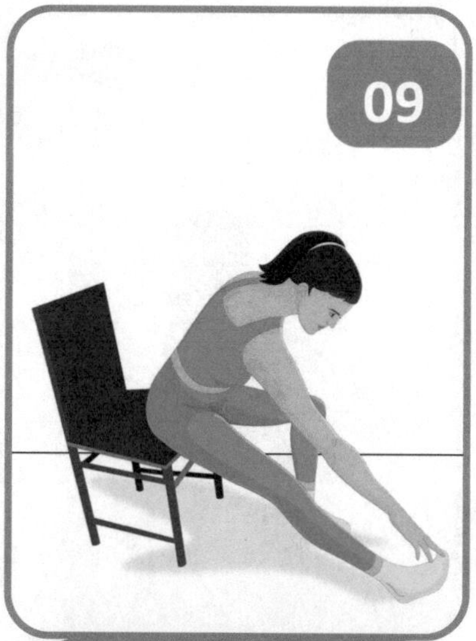

Chair
Calf Stretch

15 seconds stretch each side

Chair
Forward Fold

4 reps

Day 22 - Perform it four times

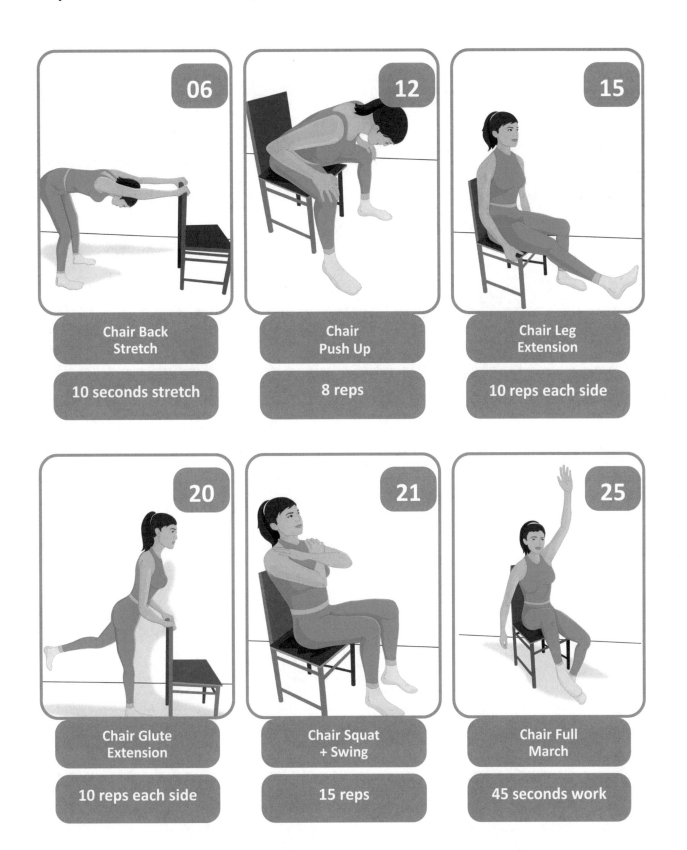

Chair Back Stretch

10 seconds stretch

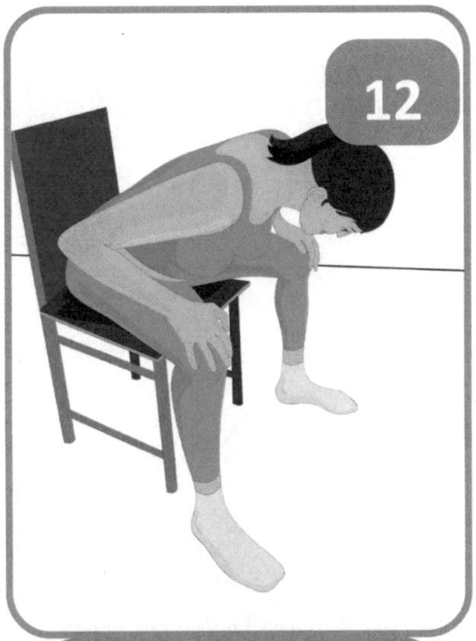

Chair Push Up

8 reps

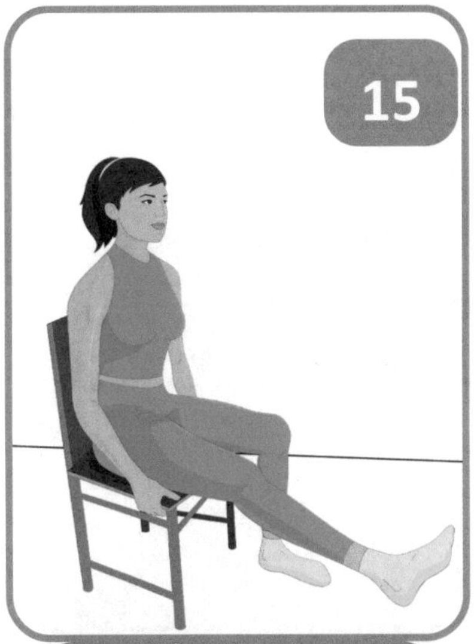

Chair Leg Extension

10 reps each side

Chair Glute Extension

10 reps each side

Chair Squat + Swing

15 reps

Chair Full March

45 seconds work

Day 23 - Perform it four times

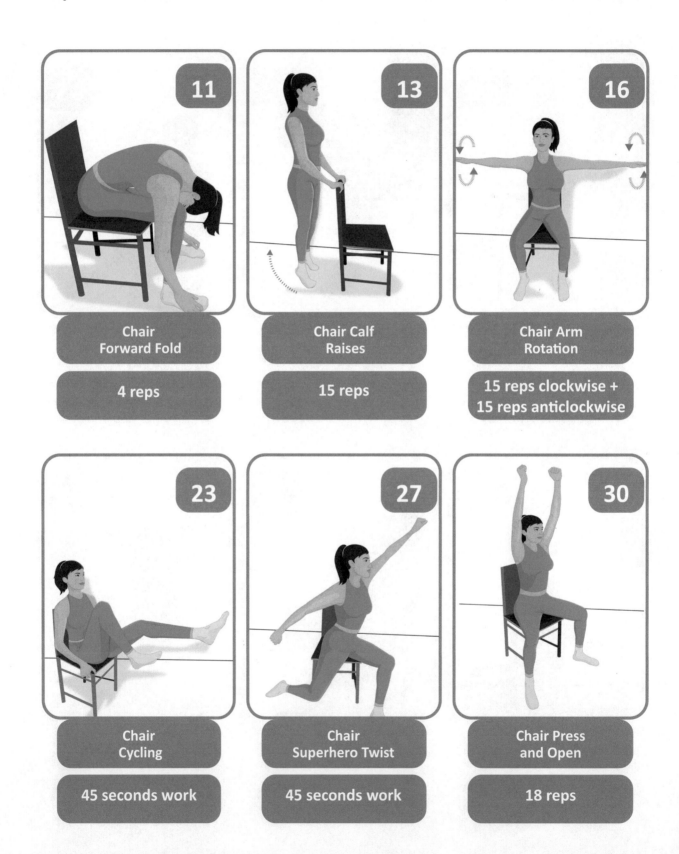

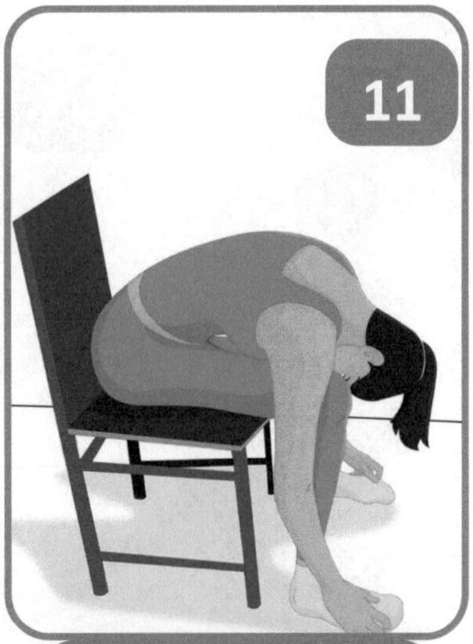

Chair Forward Fold

4 reps

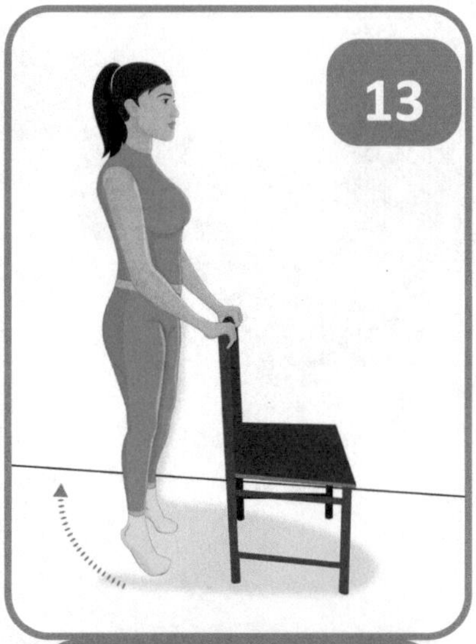

Chair Calf Raises

15 reps

Chair Arm Rotation

15 reps clockwise + 15 reps anticlockwise

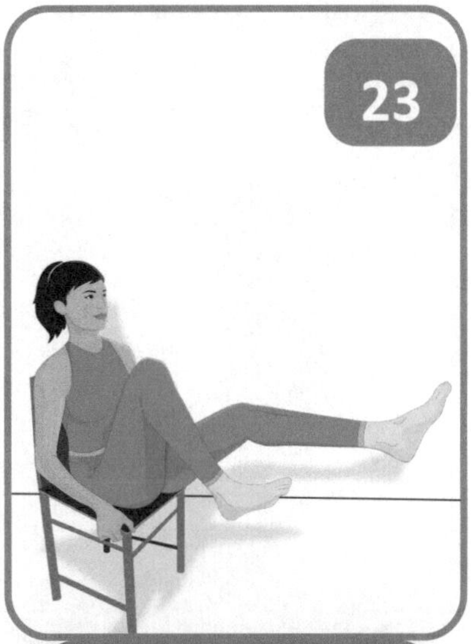

Chair Cycling

45 seconds work

Chair Superhero Twist

45 seconds work

Chair Press and Open

18 reps

Day 24 - Perform it four times

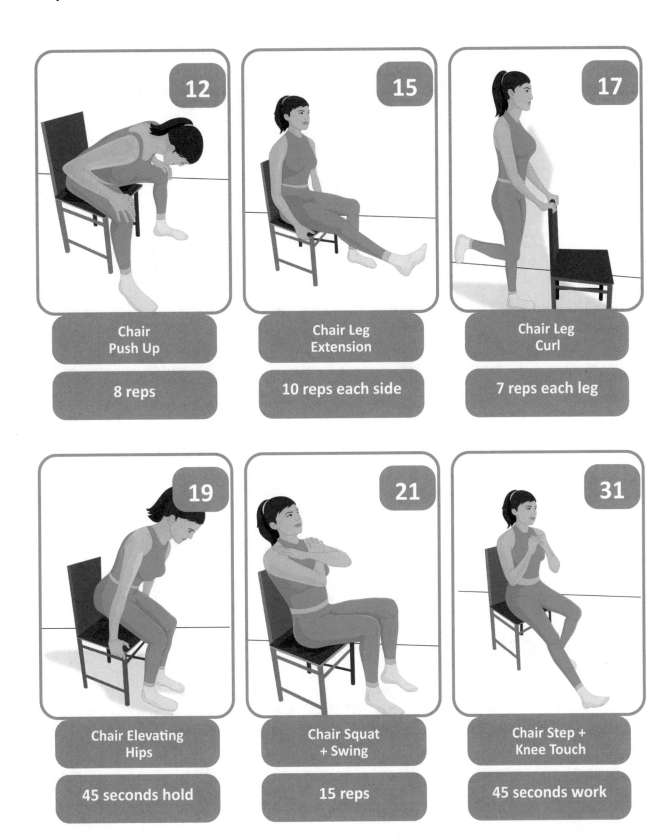

Chair
Push Up

8 reps

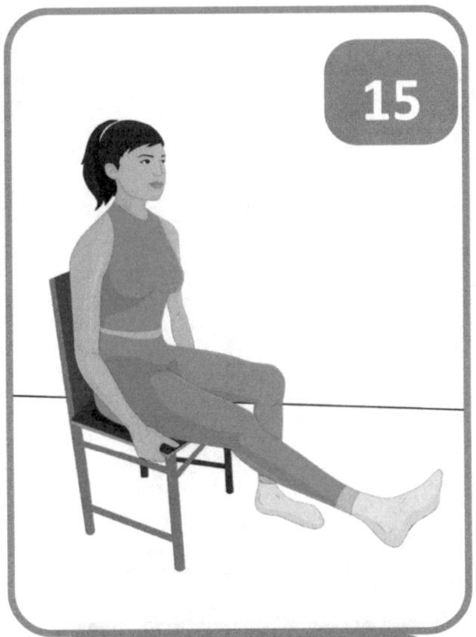

Chair Leg
Extension

10 reps each side

Chair Leg
Curl

7 reps each leg

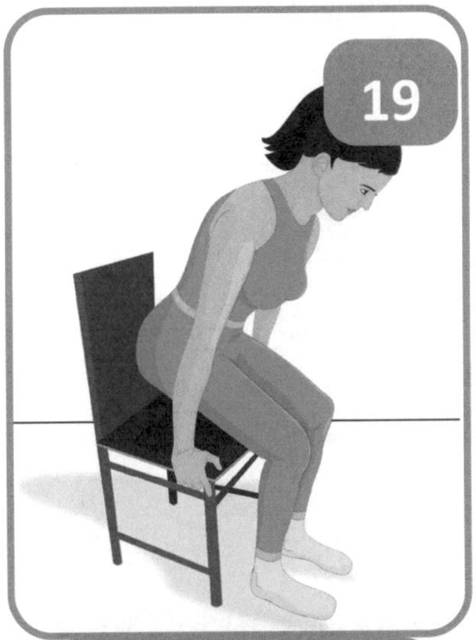

Chair Elevating
Hips

45 seconds hold

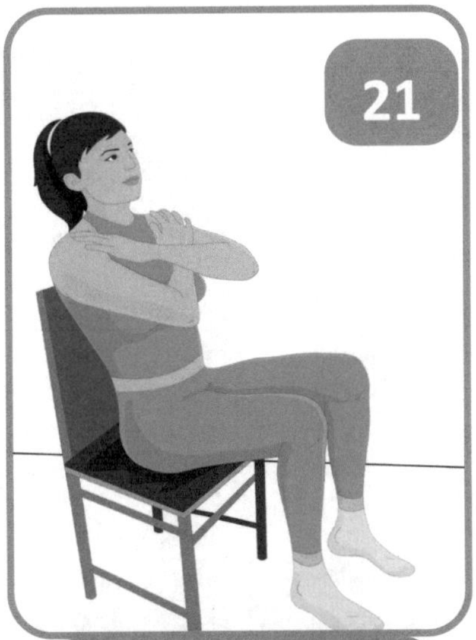

Chair Squat
+ Swing

15 reps

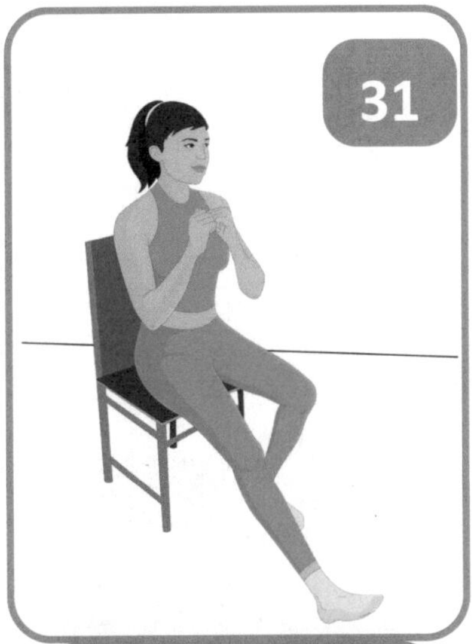

Chair Step +
Knee Touch

45 seconds work

Day 25 - Perform it four times

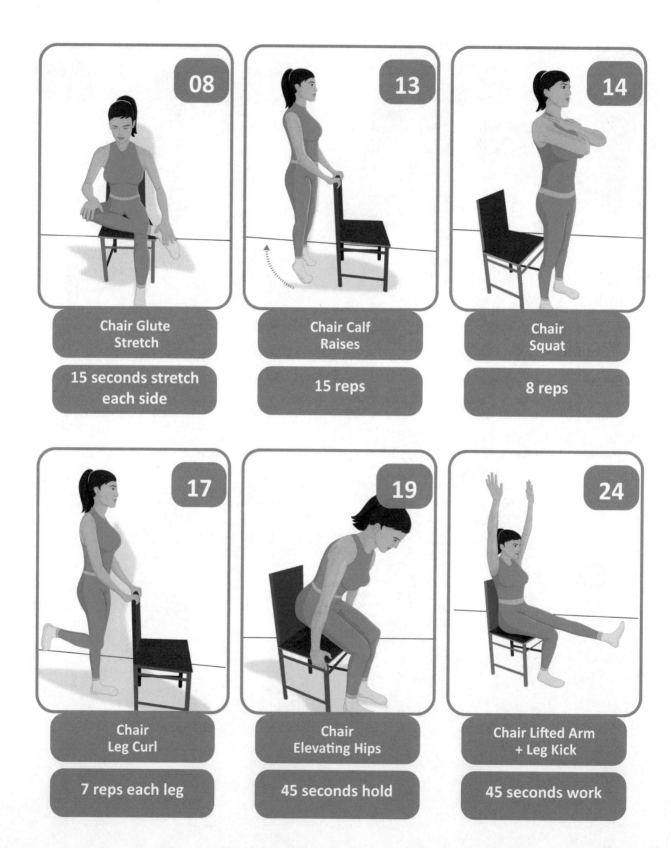

Chair Glute Stretch

15 seconds stretch each side

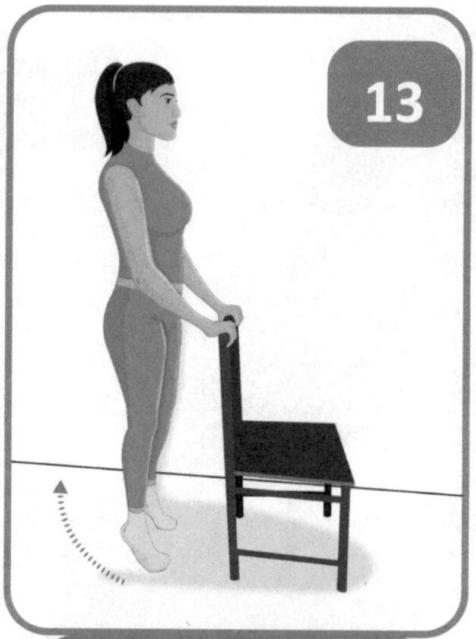

Chair Calf Raises

15 reps

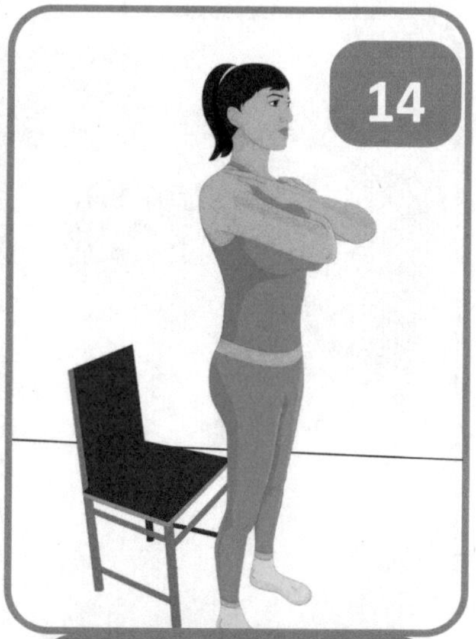

Chair Squat

8 reps

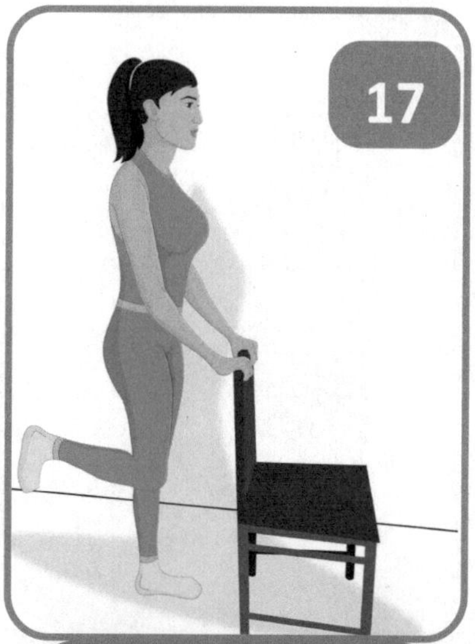

Chair Leg Curl

7 reps each leg

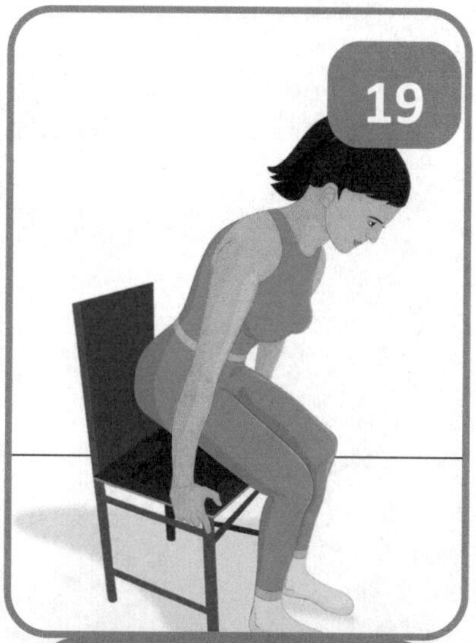

Chair Elevating Hips

45 seconds hold

Chair Lifted Arm + Leg Kick

45 seconds work

Day 26 - Perform it four times

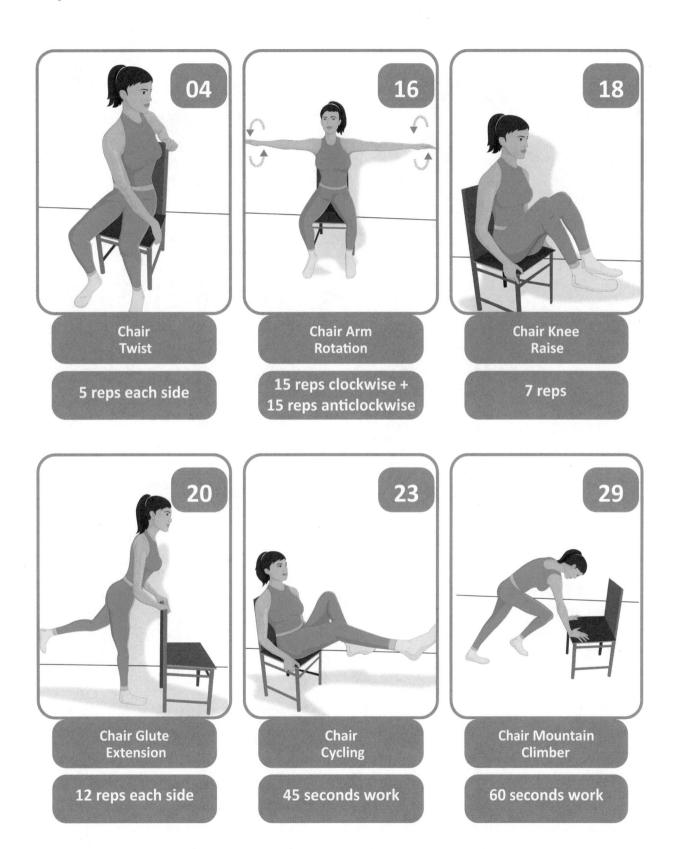

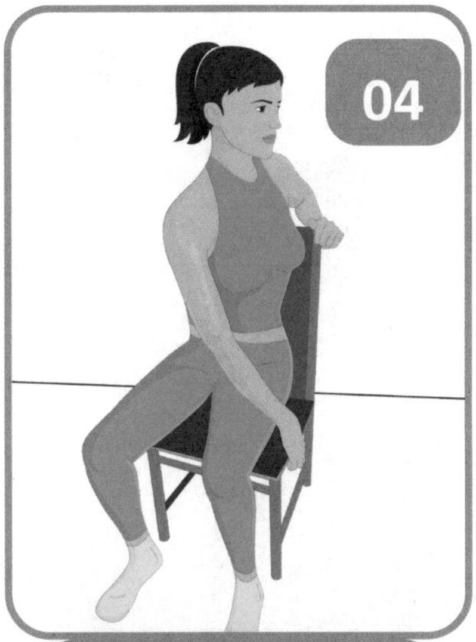

Chair Twist

5 reps each side

Chair Arm Rotation

15 reps clockwise + 15 reps anticlockwise

Chair Knee Raise

7 reps

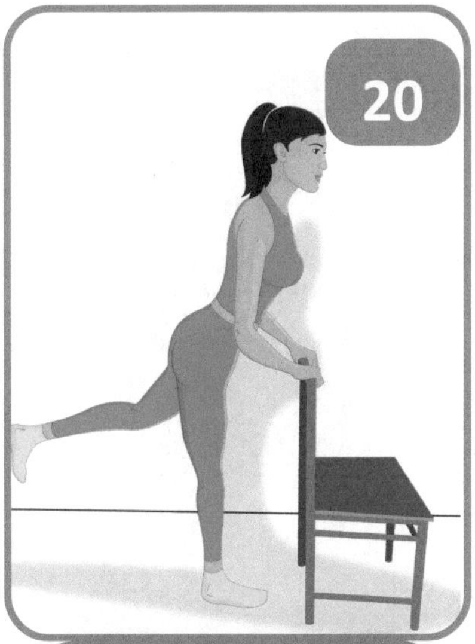

Chair Glute Extension

12 reps each side

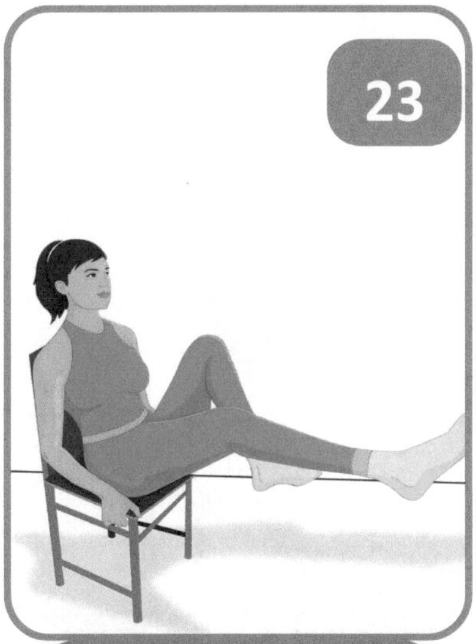

Chair Cycling

45 seconds work

Chair Mountain Climber

60 seconds work

Day 27 - Perform it four times

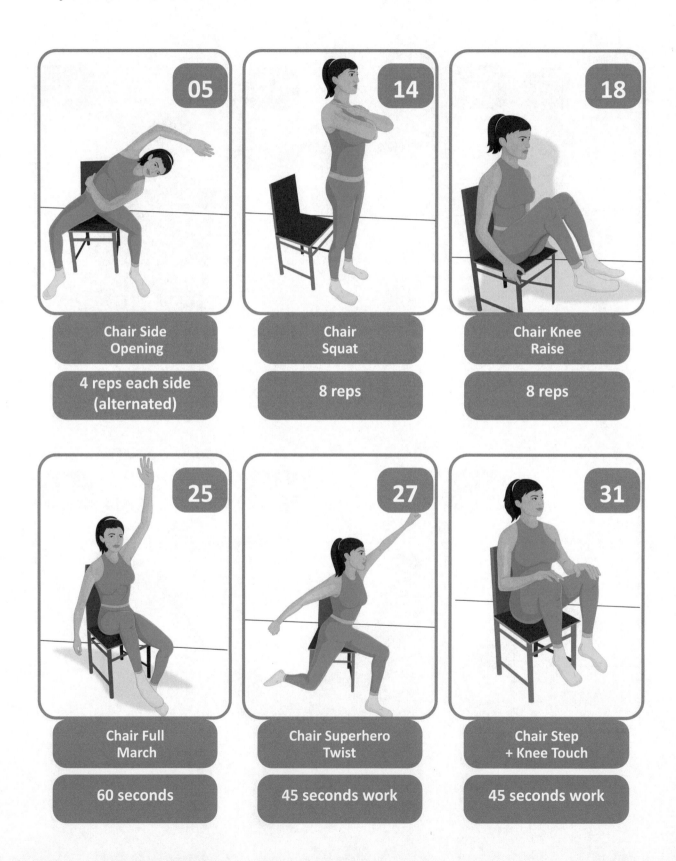

Chair Side Opening

4 reps each side (alternated)

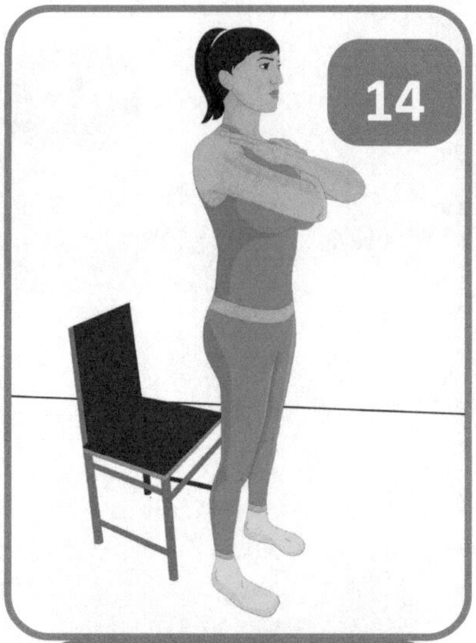

Chair Squat

8 reps

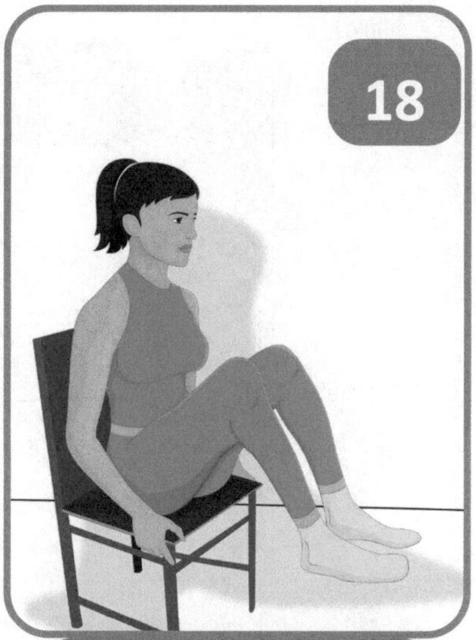

Chair Knee Raise

8 reps

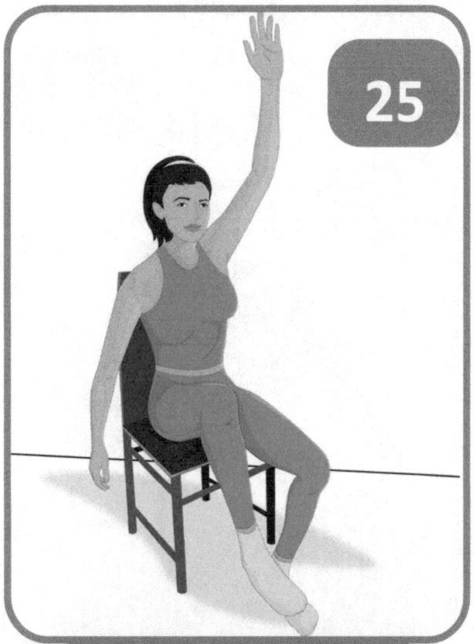

Chair Full March

60 seconds

Chair Superhero Twist

45 seconds work

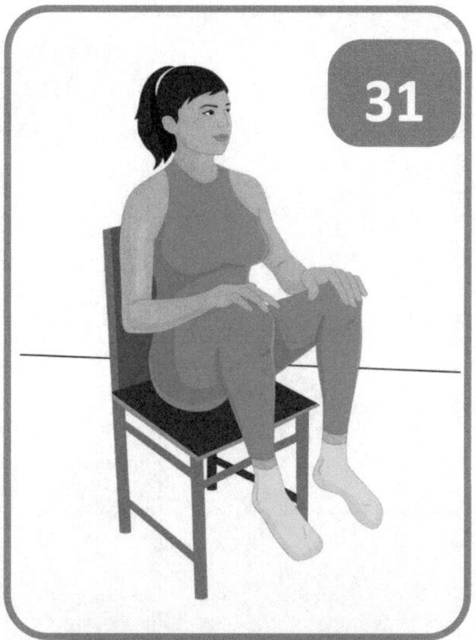

Chair Step + Knee Touch

45 seconds work

Day 28 - Perform it twice - Stretching only

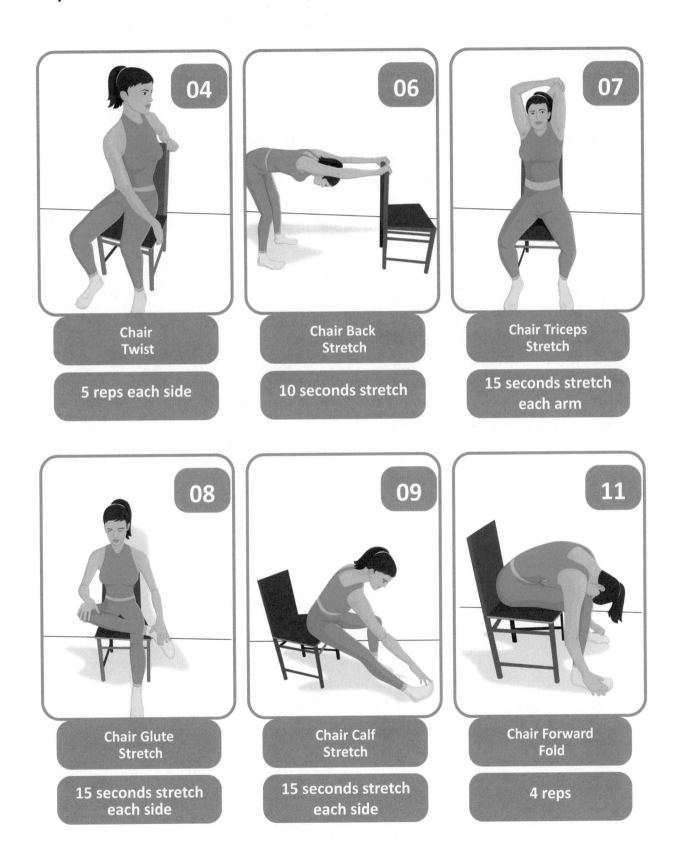

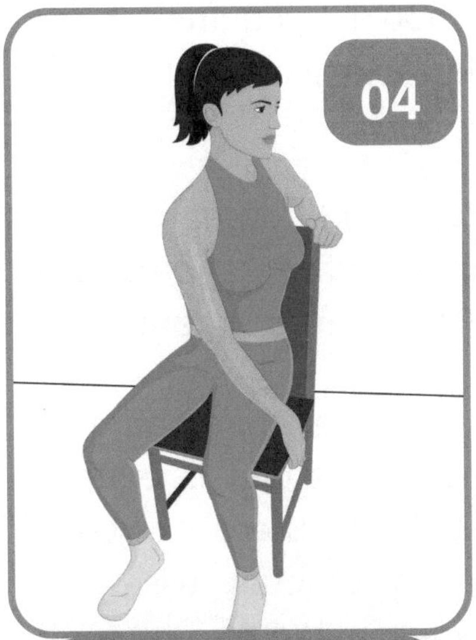

Chair Twist

5 reps each side

Chair Back Stretch

10 seconds stretch

Chair Triceps Stretch

15 seconds stretch each arm

Chair Glute Stretch

15 seconds stretch each side

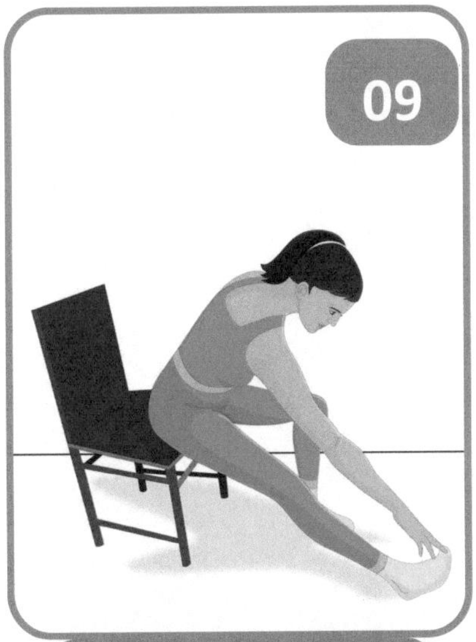

Chair Calf Stretch

15 seconds stretch each side

Chair Forward Fold

4 reps

CONCLUSION

Thank you so much for taking the time to read the book! I genuinely hope that you find the layout, illustrations, and the detailed explanations for each exercise enjoyable and informative.

I have a strong belief that incorporating these exercises and doing the 28-day challenge can truly make a positive difference in your fitness journey. I am genuinely excited for you to experience the benefits of this program.

It's important to keep in mind that while exercise is a crucial component of your fitness regimen, maintaining a balanced and nutritious diet is equally vital. Without a proper diet, all the hard work you put into these exercises may not yield the best results. So, remember to fuel your body wisely to make the most of your efforts - Simply by reducing your intake of junk food and sugar, you can make a great start!

Wishing you good health and success on your fitness journey!

See you in the next fitness book!

ABOUT ME

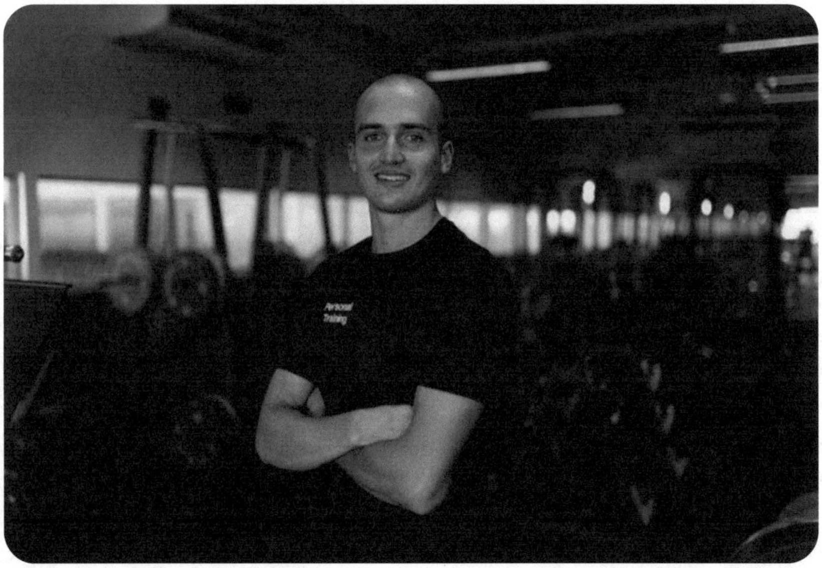

My name is Alessandro, I am Italian and lived in Milan, London, and now, Valencia, Spain. My passion for fitness started in my childhood and never stopped since then.

I am a certified Personal Trainer with years of experience in United Kingdom and Spain. I have been studying fitness articles and guides to make people fitter for years. My experience helping hundreds of people led me to write numerous books on it.

The goal is to make them healthier, more flexible, stronger, and enjoy life more.

I have been doing 1-on-1 sessions, group sessions and online coaching with people of all ages. However, I gained more experience in the last few years with people over 50 and 60. Hence why my passion in helping them skyrocketed, leasing to write guide to get to as many people as possible.

I dream of a world in which age is just a number!

It's not over yet! Scan here to receive two free eBooks.

Discover
Stress-Relief Exercises

Rediscover The Joy of
Movement and
Become Independent
Once Again

We hope you enjoy them! If you'd like to share your thoughts, it would mean the world to us. Your feedback helps us grow and create even better content for you.

Made in the USA
Columbia, SC
17 November 2024

46819439R10041